T0176470

BIOSECURITY DILEMMAS

BIOSECURITY DILEMMAS

Dreaded Diseases, Ethical Responses, and the Health of Nations

CHRISTIAN ENEMARK

Georgetown University Press / Washington, DC

Library of Congress Cataloging-in-Publication Data

Names: Enemark, Christian, author.
Title: Biosecurity dilemmas : dreaded diseases, ethical responses, and the health of nations / Christian Enemark.
Description: Washington, DC : Georgetown University Press, 2017. | Includes bibliographical references and index.
Identifiers: LCCN 2016024115 (print) | LCCN 2016040083 (ebook) | ISBN 9781626164048 (pb : alk. paper) | ISBN 9781626164031 (hc : alk. paper) | ISBN 9781626164055 (eb)
Subjects: LCSH: Biosecurity. | Biosecurity—Moral and ethical aspects. | Bioterrorism—Prevention. | Communicable diseases. | Biological arms control. | Public health—Moral and ethical aspects. | National security.
Classification: LCC JZ5865.B56 E54 2017 (print) | LCC JZ5865.B56 (ebook) | DDC 174.2/944—dc23
LC record available at https://lccn.loc.gov/2016024115

♾ This book is printed on acid-free paper meeting the requirements of the American National Standard for Permanence in Paper for Printed Library Materials.

18 17   9 8 7 6 5 4 3 2 First printing

Printed in the United States of America

Cover design by N. Putens. Cover image © Karayuschij | Dreamstime.com.

For Bree and Henry

CONTENTS

TABLES

ACKNOWLEDGMENTS

THE EARLY STAGES OF RESEARCH for this book were conducted as part of a Discovery Project on "Infectious Diseases, Security and Ethics" (no. DP0987012) funded by the Australian Research Council. For their valuable advice and encouragement, I thank my colleagues Richard Beardsworth, Huw Bennett, Madeline Carr, Campbell Craig, Alan Dupont, Mike Foley, Jonathan Herington, Rebecca Hester, Suzanne Hindmarch, Adam Kamradt-Scott, Tom Kompas, Milja Kurki, Jenny Mathers, Colin McInnes, Amy Patterson, Anne Roemer-Mahler, Simon Rushton, Jan Ruzicka, Elke Schwartz, Kamila Stullerova, and Sridar Venkatapuram. Special thanks go to Stefan Elbe, Andrew Price-Smith, and Jeremy Youde for the inspiration they have provided over many years, and to Don Jacobs for his professionalism and many courtesies. Most of all I thank my wife and son, to whom this book is dedicated.

ABBREVIATIONS

AG	Australia Group
ASM	American Society for Microbiology
ATCC	American Type Culture Collection
BSL	biosafety level
BW	biological weapons
BWC	Biological Weapons Convention
CAP	College of American Pathologists
CBM	confidence-building measure
CDC	Centers for Disease Control and Prevention
DHHS	Department of Health and Human Services
DHS	Department of Homeland Security
DSGL	Defence and Strategic Goods List (Australia)
DURC	dual-use research of concern
EO	executive order
EU	European Union
FBI	Federal Bureau of Investigation
FDA	Food and Drug Administration
GAO	Government Accountability Office
GHSA	Global Health Security Agenda
GHSI	Global Health Security Initiative
GoF	gain-of-function
ICBM	intercontinental ballistic missile
IHR	International Health Regulations
LAI	laboratory-acquired infection
MDR-TB	multidrug-resistant tuberculosis
NBACC	National Biodefense Analysis and Countermeasures Center
NIAID	National Institute of Allergy and Infectious Diseases
NIH	National Institutes of Health
NRC	National Research Council

NSABB	National Science Advisory Board for Biosecurity
PHEIC	public health emergency of international concern
PIPF	Pandemic Influenza Preparedness Framework
PPP	potential pandemic pathogen
PRP	personnel reliability program
R&D	research and development
SARS	Severe Acute Respiratory Syndrome
SNS	Strategic National Stockpile
SRA	security risk assessment
TB	tuberculosis
UN	United Nations
UNMEER	UN Mission for Ebola Emergency Response
USAMRIID	US Army Medical Research Institute for Infectious Diseases
WHA	World Health Assembly
WHO	World Health Organization
WMD	weapons of mass destruction
XDR-TB	extensively drug-resistant tuberculosis

INTRODUCTION

IN MARCH 2014 A DEADLY VIRUS was spreading across Guinea. It was the virus that causes Ebola, a form of hemorrhagic fever, and the epidemic it sparked soon became the worst of its kind on record. Within a year the disease had killed at least ten thousand people in West Africa, but this alone does not explain the enormous amount of attention that the Ebola outbreak attracted throughout the world.[1] Death can come to a person in a variety of ways, but some ways can seem far worse than others, and the possibility of dying of Ebola was terrifying to many people. The humanitarian aid organization Médecins Sans Frontières, which was deeply involved in responding to the Ebola outbreak, claimed in a 2015 report "Ebola provokes an . . . almost universal fear that is unequalled by any other disease."[2] Fear, as Daniel Deudney has observed, is "the emotion most intimately linked to security."[3] This book focuses on those dreaded diseases that governments have variously framed in security terms. These "security" diseases are often contagious but always infectious (caused by bacteria, viruses, or other microorganisms), and these two facts alone set them apart from diseases lacking a microbial cause (e.g., diabetes, stroke, and cancer). Although the latter are certainly serious health burdens in many places, the sudden outbreak of a deadly infectious disease has a greater tendency to excite the urgent attention of policy-makers concerned about national security. As this book will show, however, the adoption of a security-oriented approach to preventing or responding to disease outbreaks is not necessarily a good thing.

In a 1952 article Arnold Wolfers argued that "no policy . . . can escape becoming a subject for moral judgment . . . which calls for the sacrifice of other values, as any security policy is bound to do."[4] He highlighted, as a matter of ethical concern, the way by which, for better or for worse, "security" can manifest as a political *practice* (as distinct from a desirable state of being). When conceived in this way, security is not something that is inherently good, and the matter for judgment becomes, Is activity X a good *form* of security practice? In the name of security, many a vital project has been funded and also much money has been wasted. Appealing to security concerns can be a device not only for raising public awareness but also for maintaining secrecy; a determination to pursue security can result in the achievement of good goals as well as the perpetration of injustices. It might also be the case, moreover, that policymakers seeking to "do the right thing" encounter deep uncertainty about whether the benefit to be derived from choosing to implement a particular security practice outweighs the harm that might result from it. That is, in some situations deemed to be of security concern, a policy dilemma can arise.

The aim of *Biosecurity Dilemmas* is to highlight and explain the tension between differing values and interests that are generated or exacerbated by the practice of "biosecurity." Biosecurity is here defined as the safeguarding of populations within and among states against selected infectious disease risks. These risks include both the natural occurrence of deadly disease outbreaks and the deliberate dissemination of pathogenic microorganisms (that is, biological weapons). This book is founded on recognition of the close relationship that exists between these two areas of concern. In this way it differs from literature that addresses the security significance of only one or the other.[5] Rather, the focus has more in common with the work of authors who advance their ideas based on a comprehensive definition of biosecurity.[6] Gregory Koblentz, for example, has argued in favor of a broad definition because it helps "make explicit what would otherwise be implicit trade-offs that reduce the risk of one type of biological threat while increasing the risk of another."[7] Indeed, by highlighting these trade-offs, the processes of responding to the problem of biological weapons are potentially made more sensitive to the challenges posed by disease outbreaks of natural origin, and vice versa. And, when concerns about public health, national security, and scientific progress intersect, it is important for analysts and policymakers to be able to identify and address the tensions that erupt along the fault lines between secrecy and openness, restriction and freedom, population health and individual health, and so on. When confronting an infectious disease risk, each of these competing values will be worthy of consideration. But a "biosecurity dilemma" might arise over which values should be subordinated (at least temporarily) to others. In situations that seem to demand the protective effect of a particular biosecurity practice, the risk is that the practice taken will be more harmful than beneficial. For example, would preventing scientists from perpetrating biological attacks serve to reduce a population's overall vulnerability to infectious disease outbreaks, or would such efforts increase that vulnerability by impeding scientists' ability to make lifesaving discoveries about the organisms that cause disease?

When Jessica Stern proposed in a 2002 article that a qualitative "risk trade-off analysis" was necessary to inform policy when addressing biological weapons risks, she provided the example of its applicability also to a person "deciding whether to take aspirin for a headache, despite the increased risk of stomach upset."[8] Her concern at the time was that the US government's feverish scramble to address terrorist threats after September 11, 2001, was precluding a careful balancing of competing interests. In suggesting that the "medicine" of security policy is neither necessarily nor always good, Stern warned that the unquantifiable but "dreaded" risk of deliberate infection was possibly leading to "the design of reactive policies whose costs may exceed their benefits."[9] It was an example, perhaps, of the tendency of governments (especially democratic ones) to respond to "probability neglect"; that is, when people's emotions are intensely engaged, they are often far more concerned about dramatic risks (e.g., terrorism or an Ebola outbreak) than about statistically larger risks that are confronted in everyday life (such as car fatalities or air pollution).[10] This disproportionate concern has been found to correlate closely with a strong desire for risk reduction, including through stricter government regulation.[11] For present purposes, then, the emotion of "dread" as a political reality seems to be an important one because it goes some way to explaining why certain kinds of infectious disease risks (and not others) are made the subject of security practices.

Among the hundreds of microorganisms that are known to cause disease in humans, only a few inspire a high level of collective fear, especially in more developed countries that are less accustomed to infectious diseases posing a deadly risk. Although the names and number of these dreaded diseases cannot be definitely determined, a roundup of today's "usual suspects" would likely include anthrax, Ebola, pandemic influenza, drug-resistant tuberculosis (TB), plague, and smallpox, all of which are featured in this book. These diseases appear most frequently on various lists used for identifying government priorities for research, regulation, surveillance, and rapid response to outbreaks. For example, according to the US Centers for Disease Control and Prevention (CDC), one of the criteria for assigning a pathogenic microorganism to the "Category A" list is that it "might cause public panic and social disruption."[12] The very fact that some infectious diseases are so listed serves perhaps to confirm their fearsomeness. In any event, the dread they inspire is probably attributable to a combination of qualitative factors beyond simply the number of cases or deaths experienced or expected in an outbreak. These factors include a disease's historical reputation, its horrific symptoms, the unavailability of effective medical treatment, the apparent inability of medical science to provide a remedy at all, and the past or potential use of a disease in a biological attack. The latter might be an especially powerful factor that compounds people's visceral fear of involuntary exposure to an unfamiliar and invisible (microscopic) risk, in the sense that it seems worse to be deliberately and maliciously infected. In addition, any collective dread of infection is

continually reinforced in Western societies by a long tradition of fascinating "outbreak narratives" that have appeared in fictional literature and the performing
arts. These, in abundant ways, present opportunities for people to imagine deadly
contagion causing sudden and negative change in the social order.[13] Examples of
this narrative in literature range from Albert Camus's 1947 novel *The Plague* (an
allegory of the Nazi occupation of France) to Stephen King's *The Stand* (in which
a weaponized influenza virus kills 99 percent of the world's population). Nonlit-
erary examples range from the absurd 1954 "Dreaded Lurgi" radio play on *The
Goon Show* to Steven Soderbergh's 2011 thriller film, *Contagion*.

When populations within and among states confront a dreaded disease risk—
for example, an influenza pandemic or a biological attack involving smallpox—
governments often assume a responsibility to address the cause of that dread.
However, a strong appetite, fueled by fear, for the protection supposedly afforded
by a particular biosecurity practice should not preclude consideration of the
downsides of that practice. It is important for policymakers to be sensitive to
the possibility of doing more harm than good. Adopting a security-oriented
approach to prevent or respond to selected infectious disease risks can garner
extra resources and stronger regulatory powers for risk-reduction purposes, but
such an approach can sometimes manifest in policies and practices that are ineffective, counterproductive, and unjust. This is true for at least four overlapping
areas of policy concern: the threat of biological weapons, the risks of laboratory research on pathogenic microorganisms, the impact on societies of naturally
occurring disease outbreaks, and the effect and management of disease risks in
the context of international relations. Accordingly, parts I through IV of this
book present an analysis of four biosecurity dilemmas, drawing on ideas and
information from a range of disciplines. Of particular relevance to the discussion
of benefits and harms is the literature on the relationship between human rights
and the control of infectious diseases, on "dual-use dilemmas" encountered in
the context of scientific research, and on the shaping of international health and
security policy.[14]

Part I explores the first biosecurity dilemma, here labeled "protect or proliferate." This dilemma potentially arises from research conducted by states for
the purpose of defending against biological attacks (biodefense), and it can be
encountered at an international or domestic level. At the international level, considered in chapter 1, some biodefense efforts or technologies of one state, purportedly aimed at affording protection against microorganisms that are deliberately
disseminated, might be perceived by another state as having an offensive purpose. For example, experimentation with dissemination mechanisms for "threat
assessment" purposes could appear suspicious. If offense-defense differentiation
were extremely difficult and the suspicions of the other state drive it to engage in

the same "biodefense" activities, the result could be a proliferation of biological weapon risks and an increased likelihood of attacks while each side competed for advantage. The maintenance of a technological edge is discussed also in chapter 2, where the "protect or proliferate" dilemma is considered at the domestic level. Here the subject of concern is the potential for an increase in biological weapons risks *within* a state (vertical proliferation) as the result of an expansion of its biodefense activities. The discussion focuses on the vast biodefense program that operates in the United States: with so many people now engaged in such work, there is arguably an increased chance of a pathogenic microorganism leaking out due to a laboratory accident or being harmfully misused by a scientist.

The management of the latter risk is the subject of part II, which explores the second biosecurity dilemma: "secure or stifle." This dilemma can arise from government attempts to prevent biological attacks by regulating the conduct of pathogen research by scientists and the transfer of research-relevant materials and information. While it is true that an individual scientist could choose to misuse his or her knowledge of and access to pathogens, the overall enterprise of scientific discovery has the potential to contribute to the saving of many lives in the event of a biological attack or a natural disease outbreak. Therefore, the securing of populations against infectious disease risks can seem at once to require both the restriction and facilitation of research efforts. Chapter 3 focuses on the regulation of "laboratory biosecurity," involving the physical and personnel-based restrictions aimed at reducing the risk of laboratory insiders causing harm. These restrictions make pathogen research more difficult, expensive, and time-consuming, so the conundrum for policymakers is to determine what kind of regulation is necessary to reduce the risk of biotechnology being misused and what measures are likely instead to thwart the acquisition of knowledge applicable for health-protection purposes. In chapter 4 the discussion shifts to the fruits of laboratory-based research and whether or how these results should be shared. Of particular concern is the sharing of experimental techniques (through publication in scientific journals) that result in the creation of a microorganism more dangerous to humans than the originals (i.e., more transmissible, more virulent, more resistant to antibiotics, etc.). On the one hand, it might be argued, the mass communication of information on how a pathogen can be made more dangerous could encourage and enable the use of that information for a harmful purpose. On the other, making such findings widely available to other scientists might assist the development of new or improved measures for controlling the relevant infectious disease.

To the extent that pathogen research facilitates the availability of more and better drugs for preventing and treating infection, disease control can be undertaken without resorting to nonpharmaceutical measures. However, in circumstances where such measures are the only thing available to governments, a third kind of biosecurity dilemma can arise: "remedy or overkill." These biosecurity practices (considered in part III) are aimed at responding to rather than preventing a dreaded disease outbreak, and the discussion focuses on naturally occurring outbreaks. Even in the absence of a human enemy, a government might move to frame a natural outbreak as a matter of national security and thus claim the need to respond swiftly and aggressively. In doing so, a critical advantage might be obtained in the form of extraordinary power, effort, or resources. However, there is a risk also that such a response, implemented urgently in an atmosphere of dread, will transgress normal rules in a way that is unjust and counterproductive to public health. Chapter 5 explores the advantages and disadvantages of implementing, for the sake of national security, domestic-level "social distancing." This is a nonpharmaceutical approach to disease control that necessarily infringes on people's freedom of movement, extreme forms of which include forced isolation and mass quarantine. An assessment of these measures in chapter 5, with regard to drug-resistant TB and Ebola, respectively, is followed by an assessment of nonpharmaceutical biosecurity measures implemented at the international level. Here a "remedy or overkill" dilemma may arise in the form of border-policing practices, including prohibitions on travel between states, which restrict the cross-border flow of people who might be carrying a dreaded disease as well as people who are able to treat it.

The fourth biosecurity dilemma, "attention or neglect," is explored in part IV. It concerns the institutionalization of priority status for dreaded diseases in health policy settings. In international health-governance arrangements, and as a matter of national public health policy, it can sometimes seem difficult to achieve extra protection against certain kinds of disease risks (including biological attacks) without neglecting other health issues over the long term. At the heart of this biosecurity dilemma is the tension between policies that satisfy the greatest quantum of human need versus those that are politically feasible. Whereas the framing of some infectious diseases in security terms might attract political attention and bring certain health benefits, it might be an arrangement that promises less benefit than one whose broader humanitarian rationale might be harder politically to support over time. Chapter 7 assesses the way in which surveillance of and rapid response to some disease risks are prioritized as part of an agenda of "global health security." Although the pursuit of this agenda has the potential to protect populations in developed and developing countries alike against outbreaks with transnational reach, it arguably does less to address underlying health problems in poorer parts of the world. Finally, in chapter 8 the "attention or neglect" dilemma is considered at the level of national policy, and the discussion returns to biodefense activities within the United States. Here, the matter for judgment is whether US projects for disease surveillance (BioWatch) and pharmaceutical stockpiling (BioShield), as defenses against diseases of bioterrorism concern, are operating to the overall benefit or detriment of public health.

Throughout the book much attention is directed toward the activities of various branches of the US government because the United States is clearly in a strong position to shape the political relationship between dreaded diseases and the health of nations. The US biodefense establishment that funds and conducts pathogen research is the largest in the world, US regulations on that research are the most highly developed, and the US government is often heavily influential in the governance of international health and security affairs. Even so, *Biosecurity Dilemmas* can enlighten anyone anywhere who is interested in the politics surrounding infectious disease risks. In addition to highlighting and explaining the tensions between different interests, approaches, priorities, and purposes, the discussion also offers a number of specific policy suggestions with a view to reducing those tensions. Thus it aims to encourage critical and more integrated thinking about a broad range of biosecurity practices. Such thinking promises to improve the quality of debate and decision making at a time when deadly disease outbreaks are a great and growing concern worldwide.

NOTES

1. World Health Organization, "Ebola Situation Report—25 March 2015," March 22, 2015, http://apps.who.int/ebola/current-situation/ebola-situation-report-25-march-2015.
2. Médecins Sans Frontières, "Pushed to the Limit and Beyond: A Year into the Largest Ever Ebola Outbreak," March 23, 2015, http://www.msf.org.uk/article/ebola-pushed-to-the-limit-and-beyond-msf-report.
3. Daniel Deudney, *Bounding Power: Republican Security Theory from the Polis to the Global Village* (Princeton: Princeton University Press, 2006), 32.
4. Arnold Wolfers, "'National Security' as an Ambiguous Symbol," *Political Science Quarterly* 67, no. 4 (1952): 498.
5. See Barry Kellman, *Bioviolence: Preventing Biological Terror and Crime* (New York: Cambridge University Press, 2007); Kathleen M. Vogel, *Phantom Menace or Looming Danger?: A New Framework for Assessing Bioweapons Threats* (Baltimore: Johns Hopkins University Press, 2013); Susan Peterson, "Epidemic Disease and National Security," *Security Studies* 12, no. 2 (2002): 43–81; and Andrew T. Price-Smith, *The Health of Nations: Infectious Disease, Environmental Change, and Their Effects on National Security and Development* (Cambridge: MIT Press, 2002).
6. See Stephen J. Collier and Andrew Lakoff, "The Problem of Securing Health," in *Biosecurity Interventions: Global Health and Security in Question*, ed. Andrew Lakoff and Stephen J. Collier (New York: Columbia University Press, 2008); and David P. Fidler and Lawrence O. Gostin, *Biosecurity in the Global Age: Biological Weapons, Public Health, and the Rule of Law* (Stanford, CA: Stanford University Press, 2008).

7. Gregory D. Koblentz, "Biosecurity Reconsidered: Calibrating Biological Threats and Responses," *International Security* 34, no. 4 (2010): 108.
8. Jessica Stern, "Dreaded Risks and the Control of Biological Weapons," *International Security* 27, no. 3 (2002/03): 91.
9. Ibid., 102.
10. See Cass R. Sunstein, "Terrorism and Probability Neglect," *Journal of Risk and Uncertainty* 26, no. 2–3 (2003): 121–36.
11. Paul Slovic, Baruch Fischhoff, and Sarah Lichtenstein, "Facts and Fears: Understanding Perceived Risk," in *Societal Risk Assessment: How Safe Is Safe Enough?*, ed. Richard C. Schwing and Walter A. Albers, 181–216 (New York: Plenum, 1980), 211; World Health Organization, *World Health Report 2002: Reducing Risks, Promoting Healthy Life* (2002), 32.
12. Centers for Disease Control and Prevention, "Bioterrorism Overview," February 12, 2007, http://emergency.cdc.gov/bioterrorism/overview.asp.
13. See Priscilla Wald, *Contagious: Cultures, Carriers, and the Outbreak Narrative* (Durham, NC: Duke University Press, 2008); and Heather Schell, "Outburst! A Chilling True Story about Emerging-Virus Narratives and Pandemic Social Change," *Configurations* 5, no. 1 (1997): 96.
14. On control of infectious diseases see Margaret P. Battin, Leslie P. Francis, J. A. Jacobson, and Charles B. Smith, *The Patient as Victim and Vector: Ethics and Infectious Disease* (New York: Oxford University Press, 2009); and Stefan Elbe, "Should HIV/AIDS Be Securitized? The Ethical Dilemmas of Linking HIV/AIDS and Security," *International Studies Quarterly* 50, no. 1 (2006): 119–44. On dual-use dilemmas see Brian Rappert, *Biotechnology, Security, and the Search for Limits: An Inquiry into Research and Methods* (Basingstoke, UK: Palgrave Macmillan, 2007); and Seumas Miller and Michael J. Selgelid, *Ethical and Philosophical Consideration of the Dual-Use Dilemma in the Biological Sciences* (Springer, 2008). On international policy see Alexander Kelle, "Securitization of International Public Health: Implications for Global Health Governance and the Biological Weapons Prohibition Regime," *Global Governance* 13, no. 2 (2007): 217–35; and Adam Kamradt-Scott, *Managing Global Health Security: The World Health Organization and Disease Outbreak Control* (Basingstoke, UK: Palgrave Macmillan, 2015).

PART I
PROTECT OR PROLIFERATE

1

BIODEFENSE AND THE SECURITY DILEMMA

THE FIRST KIND OF BIOSECURITY DILEMMA under consideration here, "protect or proliferate," can arise when a government acts to defend a state's population against future biological attacks. A strong biodefense capability, based on a clear scientific understanding of pathogenic microorganisms (how they behave and how to resist them) affords a clear protective benefit. However, in some circumstances this capability can also generate pressure toward proliferation of biological weapons risks. At the domestic level (considered in chapter 2) this potential for proliferation accompanies an expansion of a state's biodefense activities to provide more people with access to pathogenic microorganisms that they could then misuse for harm. At the international level, considered in this chapter, a proliferation problem might arise if a particular biodefense activity were perceived as having an offensive rather than defensive purpose. If fear of being attacked caused one state to respond by engaging in activities that were in turn perceived by another state as offensive, the result could be a proliferation of fearsome "biodefense" activities driven by mutual suspicion. As each state sought to increase its knowledge of what it perceived to be the other's offensive capabilities, each could render itself more capable of using microorganisms for hostile purposes if it chose to do so. In this way biodefense would effectively generate an increase in the likelihood of biological weapons use; a defensive effort would worsen the threat to be defended against. Such is a problem with the 1972 Biological Weapons Convention (BWC), one goal of which is to reduce the overall likelihood of biological attacks on the grounds that these are an immoral mode of killing. Although the treaty's outlawing of biological weapons has probably made many states more reluctant to use them, this general reluctance might fade if some states continued to appear not to have a genuine moral objection to such weapons. In particular, if a state were regarded as being able to maintain an illegal offensive biological weapons program under the guise of biodefense, other states may feel they are entitled to arm themselves in like fashion. Increased moral acceptability of biological weapons, sustained by the imagined necessity of maintaining relevant technical proficiency, would then become another source of international pressure toward proliferation and use.

The protect or proliferate dilemma associated with some biodefense activities will be explored here in three sections. The first compares this particular biosecurity dilemma to a concept well established in scholarship on international relations: the security dilemma. With respect to biological weapons, this dilemma is compounded by the conceptual and empirical difficulty of characterizing these as "weapons." The second section focuses on the US government's operation of the world's largest national biodefense program, which is driven partly by US suspicions about other states' activities and partly by the threat of nonstate bioterrorism. Elements of the US program have in turn aroused the suspicions of other states. Thus the US approach to biodefense serves as a useful reference point for exploring the challenge of achieving protection without at the same time occasioning proliferation, particularly when it comes to "threat assessment" activities that investigate offensive applications of biotechnology. Finally, the chapter concludes with suggestions for some ways in which pressure toward proliferation caused by biodefense activities might be reduced. In this context it is most important for states to engage in (and be seen to be engaging in) activities that are not prone to be characterized as violations of the BWC.

THE SECURITY DILEMMA AND BIOLOGICAL WEAPONS

In his 2009 book, *Living Weapons*, Gregory Koblentz warned that, as national biological defense programs increase in number and size worldwide, "other states may perceive these activities as threatening, thereby providing a justification for initiating or continuing a BW [biological weapons] program."[1] The activities in question might not be, as a matter of fact, of a kind that are threatening or intended to threaten the state that perceives them from without. But when such a fact is difficult to verify, one state uncertain of another's capabilities and intentions is liable to err on the side of caution, assume the worst, and act to bolster its own security. The effect this security-seeking behavior has on other states—in increased concern for their own security—is conceivably unnecessary and counterproductive if the concern causes these other states to act in ways that confirm or compound prior fears. This predicament of wanting to improve one's security circumstances and running the risk of achieving the opposite is what John Herz called the "security dilemma."[2] Herz recognized the potential for states to fall victim to their uncertainty about each other's intentions once "the vicious circle of security and power accumulation is on." The tragedy he imagined was that "mutual fear of what initially may never have existed may subsequently bring about exactly that which is feared most."[3] The result of "less security all round," arrived at by a series of provocative actions that increase tension between states, is what Ken Booth and Nick Wheeler have referred to as a "security paradox," an outcome that defies the intuitive expectation that acting to improve one's security will serve actually to improve it.[4]

The international suspicion that lies at the heart of the security dilemma can sometimes be tempered by material considerations. Although the central point of the dilemma is that an increase in one state's security in turn decreases that of other states, it may be that everyone regards military capabilities that are geared toward offense as more fearsome than those that are plausibly defensive in nature. According to Robert Jervis, "when defensive weapons differ from offensive ones, it is possible for a state to make itself more secure without making others less secure."[5] That is, if weapons acquired to protect a state do not *also* afford that state the capability to attack another, and if the defense they afford has the advantage over the offense that might be offered, the security dilemma is ameliorated. Writing in 1978, Jervis highlighted short-range fighter aircraft and anti-aircraft missiles as two examples of capabilities more useful for defense than for offense. He observed that these "can be used to cover an attack" and "can advance with the troops," yet they are unable to "reach deep into enemy territory."[6] Likewise, Jervis observed that citizen militias lend themselves more to defense than to attacks on foreign territories because they "lack both the ability and the will for aggression," whereas "mobile heavy guns" are characterized as "particularly valuable to a state planning an attack."[7]

In other circumstances and in the context of other capabilities, however, a state might judge that an offense-defense distinction cannot plausibly and safely be drawn. The need to act out of fear would then continue to be felt, so the security dilemma would remain. Some military capabilities can indeed appear to be equally applicable to offensive and defensive actions. For example, prior to World War I, Britain's maintenance of a large navy capable of protecting shipping lanes was also perceived as menacing "any other state with a coast that could be raided, trade that could be interdicted, or colonies that could be isolated."[8] In the case of intercontinental ballistic missiles (ICBMs) bearing nuclear warheads, deep uncertainty exists about an offensive capability that is supposedly elementally defensive; a state's *defense* relies on deterring nuclear-armed enemies from attacking by threatening a nuclear *attack* as punishment. Thus the acquisition of more ICBMs, ostensibly to improve a state's ability to defend itself, is also readily the subject of fear by states whose cities would be targeted for retaliation. According to Booth and Wheeler, it is precisely the status of these weapons as "inherently ambiguous symbols" that materially establishes the security dilemma.[9] In the case of biological weapons, there can be profound ambiguity owing to the underlying technology's applicability to civilian as well as military purposes. The challenge, then, is to discern, amid the expanse of legitimate (health-protective) uses of technologies associated with pathogenic microorganisms, the intention and preparedness to use "dual-use" biotechnology offensively.

When thinking about the security dilemma, the problem with biological weapons is that, in practical terms, they are not really "weapons." A state is able to observe, judge, and react to another state's acquisition of something that is an item (a submarine, a tank, or a missile), but biological weapons are processes rather than items. Thus it is unhelpful to think of a state as *possessing* biological weapons and more accurate to think of it being in a *position* to threaten or perpetrate a biological attack. The degree of a state's proximity to that position, in terms of technical capability and intent, is the critical issue because it makes no sense in the biological realm to contemplate simply the possession or nonpossession of weapons. Whereas a rifle is always a weapon whether someone uses it or not, a pathogenic microorganism is a weapon only when it is used as such. The process of *wielding* the weapon is what counts, and that process might work as follows: a pathogenic microorganism is chosen, then cultured and produced in large quantities through a fermentation process, then inserted into a delivery mechanism such as a spray device, and then disseminated in such a way that it survives meteorological conditions on its way to infecting and sickening human targets. The closer a state is to being able to carry out such a process, the closer it is to being in a position to threaten other states. Even so, that state could also claim that it has placed itself in exactly that position only for the purpose of fully understanding the nature of the threat it faces or might face from other states. The difficulty, however, of experimenting with offensive applications of biotechnology and of claiming that doing so serves a defensive purpose is that it puts the offense-defense distinction under great pressure. If the only thing that distinguishes a biodefense program from a biological weapons program is the operator's intent, other states might take action to prepare for a sudden change of mind (by investigating the offensive capabilities they fear). Security dilemmas in combination could then lead to a security paradox: more offensive know-how all around and more danger of biological attacks against more states.

Collective concern about such an eventuality provided much impetus for the entry into force (as international law) of the Biological Weapons Convention in 1975. The first treaty designed to outlaw an entire category of weapons, the BWC was intended to address the problem of proliferation by achieving universal and permanent disarmament. Specifically, the BWC addressed development, production, stockpiling, acquisition, and retention, because member states were "determined for the sake of all mankind, to *exclude completely the possibility* of bacteriological (biological) agents and toxins being used as weapons" (emphasis added).[10] Such a determination, while admirable and ambitious, nevertheless had to be made subject to a definition of the "weapon" problem that allowed for the dual applicability (offensive and defensive) of relevant materials, technologies, and practices. Thus Article I of the BWC provides:

> Each State Party to this Convention undertakes never in any circumstances to develop, produce, stockpile, or otherwise acquire or retain:
>
> (1) Microbial or other biological agents, or toxins whatever their origin or method of production, of types and in quantities that have no justification for prophylactic, protective or other peaceful purposes;
> (2) Weapons, equipment, or means of delivery designed to use such agents or toxins for hostile purposes or in armed conflict.[11]

The language of this provision will be assessed later in this chapter, but for now it suffices to highlight the words "justification for prophylactic, protective or other peaceful purposes." This phrase effectively allows the continuation of the enormous amount of work with biological agents (microorganisms) that is carried out in and by states worldwide for biomedical research and for clinical and public health purposes. Article I of the BWC also renders legitimate many of the activities—those that are clearly benign—that are or might be conducted as part of a state's biodefense program. For example, researching, developing, and acquiring pharmaceutical resources to prevent or treat known infectious diseases (e.g., antibiotics, antivirals, antitoxins, and vaccines) is a measure aimed directly at reducing the human cost of an infectious disease outbreak (of deliberate or nondeliberate origin).

Other activities are less easy to square with the language of the BWC, and it is these that are prone to cause a security dilemma. Of particular concern, in terms of generating horizontal (international) proliferation pressure, are biodefense projects conducted for "threat assessment" purposes. Investigating possible offensive applications of pathogenic microorganisms so as to determine appropriate countermeasures does appear, at first, eminently sensible. Arguably, in order to develop defenses against a future biological attack it is fundamentally necessary to understand such things as the underlying mechanisms for a microorganism's pathogenicity, the way in which it evades the human immune system or acquires resistance to antibiotics, and ways in which it might be deliberately dispersed. An understanding of these factors is also, however, exactly what would be required in order to carry out a biological attack. If one state suspected that ill intent lay behind a second state's proficiency with dispersal technology especially, it might likewise decide to inform itself of offensive possibilities. A security dilemma will have arisen: Should that state, seeking protection, run the risk of frightening other states into biological proliferation? It is a dilemma well illustrated by the experience of the United States.

US BIODEFENSE AND THE PROBLEM OF SUSPICION

In 1969 US president Richard Nixon announced that his country would unilaterally abandon biological warfare as a military option. The decision gave a huge boost to the norm against deliberately spreading disease and laid the political groundwork for the BWC to entrench the norm in international law. When the convention was later being negotiated, many states regarded biological weapons as having little military utility anyway, and this might have led to a belief that cheating on a ban would yield no significant advantage to the cheater.[12] In any event, the BWC did have the effect of making it politically more difficult to establish or maintain a biological weapons program. A concern that the utility of such a program could increase in the future did remain, so some states that eventually signed on to the BWC continued to pursue defensive capabilities, just in case. Because the Cold War superpowers could not agree on incorporating a compliance verification mechanism into the BWC, some defensive efforts themselves soon became a source of mutual suspicion and proliferation pressure. Did those efforts involving biological materials and related technologies truly have a *"justification for prophylactic, protective or other peaceful purposes"*? It appears the Soviet Union thought it unsafe to assume as much about US biodefense activities. Rather, Nixon's 1969 decision was seen as a signal that the Americans would switch to carrying on biological research for offensive purposes in secret. In his 1999 memoir *Biohazard*, Soviet defector Ken Alibek reflected,

> We didn't believe a word of Nixon's announcement. Even though the massive U.S. biological munitions stockpile was ordered to be destroyed, and some twenty-two hundred researchers and technicians lost their jobs, we thought the Americans were only wrapping a thicker cloak around their activities.[13]

This suspicion of US cheating, coupled with a desire to match or outpace US progress on biological weapons research, drove the Soviet Union to cheat too. In 1973 (the year following the opening of the BWC for signature) the Soviet government established Biopreparat, which, from the outside, appeared to be a state-owned pharmaceutical complex developing vaccines for the civilian market.

However, soon after the fall of the Soviet Union it was revealed that Biopreparat was a military-funded program for developing new types of biological weapons.[14] This revelation confirmed US suspicions, but it was extremely rare in that regard. In the years since, although suspicions about other states have arisen or persisted, the dual-use nature of technology associated with pathogenic microorganisms has made it difficult to know for sure whether the BWC is being violated or not. It is a difficulty evidenced, for example, by the findings of a 2015 report by the US State Department addressing "BWC-related compliance questions" regarding five BWC member states—China, Iran, North Korea, Pakistan, and Russia—as well as the "biological warfare (BW)-related activities" of two non-member states—Egypt and Syria.[15] The most striking feature of the report is the use of language that reflects deep uncertainty regarding the marrying of technical capabilities with offensive intentions. The State Department reported that during the preceding twelve months, "China engaged . . . in biological activities with *potential* dual-use applications," and available information "did not indicate" that Egypt or Pakistan were "engaged in activities prohibited by the BWC."[16] Iran continued to engage in "dual-use activities with BW applications," but it was "*unclear* if these activities were conducted for purposes inconsistent with the BWC" (emphasis added). The report noted that "North Korea *may* still *consider* the use of biological weapons as an option," and that it remained "*unclear* . . . whether Syria would *consider* the use of biological weapons as a military option" (emphasis added). As for Russia, the finding was that "entities" there "remained engaged in dual-use, biological activities" and that it was "unclear" whether these activities were BWC-compliant.

The obvious concern here was the unavailability of information that would allay or reduce suspicion about these states' activities. The US government was not satisfied that Russia, for example, had documented a complete dismantling of the Soviet Union's "past offensive program of biological research and development."[17] With the possibility left open that such a program in fact exists in Russia and in other states, there is thus some justification for US biodefense efforts to be pursued on a just-in-case basis. Such efforts are also driven by concerns about bioterrorism perpetrated by nonstate actors, but either way the problem remains that certain biodefense activities could end up contributing to a biological weapons problem worthy of ever-greater concern. If uncertainty about the true purpose of such activities drives other states in turn to increase and improve their own technical capabilities, the result could be a dangerous spiral of mutual suspicion and horizontal proliferation. There is a security imperative, therefore, for any government to be sensitive to the way in which its own biodefense activities may be externally perceived. That is, to avoid arousing international suspicion, it is not enough for a state to be self-confident on the question of BWC compliance. Rather, this area of biosecurity practice requires the exercise of "security dilemma sensibility." According to Booth and Wheeler, this is the ability of an international actor to understand the role that fear might play in others' attitudes and behaviors, including "the role that one's own actions may play in provoking that fear."[18]

In the case of the United States, the most fearsome biodefense activities, which carry the greatest proliferation risk, are those that fall under the category of "threat assessment." In accordance with National Security Decision Memorandum 35, issued by National Security Advisor Henry Kissinger on November 25, 1969, the United States interprets its responsibilities under the BWC as permitting "research into those offensive aspects of bacteriological/biological agents necessary to determine what defensive measures are required."[19] The memorandum did not specify what types of research were justified for defensive purposes, but Kissinger's successor Brent Scowcroft issued a second memorandum in 1975 authorizing activities that the President had determined to be for protective or other peaceful purposes. These activities included "vulnerability studies and research, development and testing of equipment and devices such as protective masks and clothing, air and water filtration systems, detection, warning and identification devices, and decontamination systems" and "biomedical or other research for the purpose of increasing human knowledge and not intended for weapons development."[20] As of 1989, according to congressional testimony in May of that year by the then-commander of the US Army Medical Research Institute for Infectious Diseases (USAMRIID), research to increase the virulence of pathogens, to stabilize biological agents, and on dissemination methods was officially regarded as prohibited by the BWC.[21] Also, all work conducted under the Defense Department's Biological Defense Research Program was at that point in time unclassified (although research results that were deemed to impinge on national security could later be classified).[22] By the early 1990s a shift in the US government's approach to biodefense was under way, and a number of government agencies would soon afterward undertake research in exactly the areas cited previously by USAMRIID's former commander. This change was prompted initially by the revelation that the Soviet Union had been secretly pursuing a biological weapons program in violation of the BWC. Political concern inside the United States then deepened when it was discovered that Iraq, too, had been violating the convention. After the 1995 chemical attack on the Tokyo subway by members of the Aum Shinrikyo cult, it was learned that Aum had earlier attempted to use biological weapons, which served as a reminder of the security threat posed by nonstate actors. Thereafter, the US government perceived the need to not only redouble its existing biodefense efforts but also explore new areas and conduct some activities secretly.

When secret projects conducted during the late 1990s were later revealed by *New York Times* investigators, the world at large had occasion to consider whether these biodefense activities were geared more toward offense than defense. One of the projects, code-named Project Jefferson, involved experiments to reproduce the results of Russian research (published in the journal *Vaccine* in 1997) that had created a vaccine-resistant strain of *Bacillus anthracis* (anthrax) bacteria. The researchers had inserted genes from *Bacillus cereus* into *Bacillus anthracis*, making the latter highly lethal against hamsters inoculated with Russia's standard anthrax vaccine.[23] In Project Jefferson the aim was to produce small quantities (one gram or less) of this modified anthrax bacteria.[24] But was this effort, to use the words of Article I of the BWC, the production of biological agents "of type and in quantities" that had "no justification for prophylactic, protective or other peaceful purposes"? Or was the research justified because Jefferson produced only a tiny quantity of a type of biological agent that already existed (inside a Russian laboratory) as a risk to human health? The latter explanation is the more plausible, so Jefferson was probably BWC-compliant. Of greater concern, however, was Project Clear Vision, which involved building and testing a Soviet-modeled bomblet for dispersing bacteria from 1997 to 2000.[25] A number of these bomblets were reportedly filled with simulant "pathogens" (unable to cause disease) and tested for their dissemination characteristics and reliability under different atmospheric conditions. Experiments in a wind tunnel revealed how the bomblets, after being released from a warhead, would fall on targets.[26] Here, the issue (to be explored later) was whether the United States had produced a "means of delivery" in violation of the BWC.

The *New York Times* revelations occurred just a few months after an official announcement in July 2001 that the United States would not support a legal instrument for verifying member states' compliance with the BWC. In combination, these events fueled suspicion on the part of some observers that the US government likely had other dubious "biodefense" activities it wanted to hide.[27] However, any international opprobrium was quickly overshadowed by the terrorist attacks that occurred on September 11, 2001. These, and the subsequent biological attacks using anthrax-laced envelopes, confirmed President George W. Bush in his view that technological superiority, more than international law, should be America's pathway to national security. Effort and expenditure on US biodefense boomed, and the nature and intensity of threat assessment projects became all the more capable of stimulating fear in other states. The National Biodefense Analysis and Countermeasures Center (NBACC) was established under the new Department of Homeland Security (DHS), and in 2004 its deputy director delivered an alarming presentation at a Defense Department workshop on pest management. In that presentation the DHS official revealed that one of his center's research units intended to pursue a range of topics including "aerosol dynamics," "novel packaging," "novel delivery of threat," "genetic engineering," and "red teaming" (a reference to exercises modeling an enemy's anticipated modes of attack). The official summarized NBACC's "threat assessment" task areas using a series of verbs: "acquire, grow, modify, store, stabilize, package, disperse."[28] Such language is identical to language that would describe the operation of a biological weapons program and the process of perpetrating a biological attack. Outside observers would have hoped that this presentation by a US official was merely a clumsy misrepresentation of American activities that are really undertaken for peaceful purposes, but there is additional information on which other states could reasonably base a suspicion of offensive US intent. Particularly worrisome are US biodefense activities that, like Project Clear Vision, appear to bring the "biological" overly close to the "weapon."

Although research into pathogen dispersal mechanisms can inform the design or improvement of protective bodysuits and devices for detecting airborne microorganisms, it is equally the case that such research could guide the planning and execution of a biological attack. As noted in a 1998 report from the office of the US under secretary of defense for acquisition and technology: "Stabilization and dispersion are *proliferation concerns* because these technologies increase the efficacy of biological agents" (emphasis added).[29] The US government itself tends mostly to employ dispersion technologies on a small scale, inside laboratories, when using live pathogenic microorganisms. In large-scale outdoor experiments, only "simulants" (live nonpathogens or killed pathogens) are used. A 2000 report by the US Department of Energy revealed that, since 1992, the US Army had been operating two aerosol test chambers at its Edgewood Arsenal in Maryland. The chambers, which were reportedly being used for "studying explosive and nonexplosive means of delivery of dangerous microorganisms as aerosols," were 70 cubic meters and 155 cubic meters in size.[30] A much larger chamber (at 200 cubic meters) later commenced operation at the Army's Dugway Proving Ground in Utah in 2013.[31] The Whole System Live Agent Test Chamber facility is intended to "allow scientists and test officers to control temperature . . . relative humidity . . . and wind speed control . . . to simulate various climatic conditions," and it can generate "threat-representative aerosolized wet and dry biological warfare agents."[32]

Beyond the aerosolization of pathogenic microorganisms, US biodefense research also includes the use of various uncontained spaces to explore possibilities for dispersal of biological material. For example, among the "Tunnel Dissemination Systems" at Dugway, the Joint Ambient Breeze Tunnel features "a dissemination gate and overhead, four-zone Sono-Tek nozzle array, while dissemination carts provide maneuverability for precision set-up of aerosol cloud generation." Here, "portable liquid and dry dissemination systems may be operated for specific tests to replicate an attack (e.g., covert backpack attack), including electric Micronair sprayers and E2 sprayers, Skil® blowers, and puff disseminators." When a Skil® blower is used to release "5 to 10 grams" of a "dry powder simulant" it creates "a concentration of 5,000 to 20,000 particles per liter inside a tunnel."[33] The Lothar Salomon Test Facility, also at Dugway, includes the use of "simulants" in "outdoor studies" in order to "develop/validate aerosol particle dispersion models to enhance countermeasure efficacy."[34] For example, simulants used in a 2005 field trial of the Joint Biological Standoff Detection System included a "dry killed vaccine strain of *Bacillus anthracis* [anthrax]" and a "wet killed vaccine strain . . . of *Yersinia pestis* [plague]."[35] The trial included one late-night dissemination of 20 grams of dry anthrax simulant at a "target range" of 1.2 km, another 20-gram dissemination at a range of 2.6 km, and dissemination of 3.5 liters and 7.0 liters of plague simulant at a target range of 1.2 km and 7.0 km, respectively.[36]

Two assumptions drive such experimentation: that the detection systems being tested would be able to detect the dispersal of living bacteria as well as dead ones and that the dispersal mechanisms used to challenge those systems would deliver both kinds of material to the target in much the same way. It follows that the operator of the dispersal mechanisms would need only to fill them with real pathogens in order to be in a position to perpetrate a real biological attack. For this very reason, though, the US government itself would likely take a dim view of similar aerosolization and dispersal capabilities in the hands of another state. For example, when a 2005 State Department report concluded that "China maintains some elements of an offensive BW capability in violation of its BWC obligations," it explained:

> From 1993 to the present, [Chinese] military scientists have published in open literature the results of studies of aerosol stability of bacteria, models of infectious virus aerosols, and detection of aerosolized viruses. . . . Such advanced biotechnology techniques could be applicable to the development of offensive BW agents and weapons.[37]

Logically, an identical claim could be leveled against the United States for some of the techniques described earlier, and so China could today find itself facing a biosecurity dilemma: protect or proliferate? Suspicious of US intentions, China could decide to engage in similar activities in order to "assess" the threat, but US suspicions of Chinese intentions here could in turn perpetuate a competition to acquire more and better knowledge of how a biological attack could be conducted. A tragic possibility, then, is that neither state would in fact be interested in perpetrating biological attacks against the other but reciprocal fear would propel research activities and deepen their mutual insecurity. To reduce the likelihood and impact of such a situation, greater openness and trust between states is required, and this much could indeed be said about a multitude of circumstances encountered in international affairs. For present purposes, though, the specific requirements for reducing biological proliferation pressure seem to be disclosure by individual states of more information about their biodefense activities in general and avoidance altogether of the large-scale use of microbe-dispersal systems.

IMPROVING TRANSPARENCY AND BUILDING CONFIDENCE

One perspective of international politics is that, because intentions are ultimately unknowable, "states worried about their survival must make worst-case assumptions about their rivals' intentions."[38] On the issue of "knowability," however, a more plausible observation might be that states experience *degrees* of ignorance at any given time. To a greater or lesser extent, information obtained or received can shed light on whether, for example, a state has hostile or peaceful intentions toward others. Therefore, rather than always being resigned to acting on worst-case assumptions, states could exercise the option to take steps to "reduce uncertainty about each other's intentions and thus fear."[39] Sometimes a state might be able to reduce the degree of its own ignorance unilaterally. For example, after the 2003 US invasion of Iraq, which was in part an attempt at forced disarmament, the US government took steps to improve its ability to make well-informed assessments about the material capabilities of other states. The Commission on the Intelligence Capabilities of the United States Regarding Weapons of Mass Destruction stated in its 2005 report: "The Intelligence Community seriously misjudged the status of Iraq's biological weapons program."[40] Accordingly, it recommended "better collaboration between the intelligence and biological science communities."[41] The US director of national intelligence responded by, inter alia, establishing a Biological Sciences Expert Group, composed of nongovernment scientists who are paid annual retainers to review the scientific validity of intelligence assessments.[42] Such a measure might well reduce the likelihood of the US government again forming overblown suspicions about biological weapons "possession" by another state, but the greater part of the suspicion-reduction challenge is international in scope. That is, due to security dilemma dynamics, the reduction of US suspicion is closely tied to the reduction of suspicion about the United States.

In 1983, when US defense secretary Caspar Weinberger announced his country's Strategic Defense Initiative, he asserted that the Soviets had "no need to worry" about US plans for missile defense because "they know perfectly well that we will never launch a first strike on the Soviet Union."[43] The Soviets knew no such thing. Rather, Weinberger arrogantly assumed that US actions were above suspicion. In 2005 another US politician, Senate majority leader Bill Frist, displayed a similar lack of awareness about the security dilemma when he called for "an unprecedented effort—a Manhattan Project for the 21st century—not with the goal of creating a destructive new weapon, but to defend against destruction wreaked by infectious disease and biological weapons."[44] Frist's explanation of "the goal" was scarcely reassuring compared to his alarming evocation of America's development and first-use of nuclear weapons. Four years previously, in written testimony to the US Senate Committee on Foreign Relations, Nobel laureate Joshua Lederberg had warned, "We [Americans] have to be careful to behave ourselves fully consistently with abhorrence at the idea of using disease as a weapon." The "particular dilemma," as he saw it, was "how to study the BW threats in detail, how to develop vaccines and other countermeasures, without attracting . . . accusations [of breaching the BWC]." Thus, although Frist might have been justified in later advocating the pursuit of biodefense on a greater scale, Lederberg was concerned with the need also to "develop models of entrusted transparency . . . for assurance to global publics, and to be certain there are no careless projects oblivious to the reputational or physical harm they could inflict on our polity."[45]

One way to short-circuit the mutual suspicion and reduce the proliferation risk associated with biodefense programs might be to establish an international regime for verifying states' compliance with the BWC. For more than forty years, however, BWC verification has been an elusive goal, not least because of the tendency of many governments to assume that security is enhanced by secrecy. Prior to 2001, BWC member states had been negotiating a legally binding verification protocol for the convention. Broadly speaking, greater confidence in states' compliance was to be gained by declaration of facilities with the potential to engage in research and production relevant to biological weapons, routine and unannounced visits to such facilities, and investigation of suspicious disease outbreaks. The negotiations quickly unraveled after mid-2001 when the US government announced it would not support a draft verification scheme.[46] The basis for this decision was a concern (shared by some other states) that opening national facilities to international inspection teams would compromise confidential military and commercial information. Nevertheless, at subsequent BWC meetings and review conferences the idea of a verification regime has continued to receive strong support from influential states. At a meeting in Geneva, Switzerland, in August 2015 the Chinese government warned, "Due to the long-standing lack of a legally binding protocol of the Convention . . . activities for the research and development of bio-offensive capabilities have become more secret and concealed, with the possibility for the evil of biological weapons to reappear in the world."[47] Russia, too, has insisted that a verification protocol is needed because, according to one senior official, "ordinary transparency measures, with all their importance and usefulness, cannot give such certainty."[48] The "ordinary" measures referred to are the confidence-building measures (CBMs) originally agreed to at the Second Review Conference in 1986, the original purpose of which was "to prevent or reduce the occurrence of ambiguities, doubts, and suspicions."[49]

While ever the US government continues to oppose a verification regime, the political reality is that the CBMs stand as the primary mechanism by which BWC member states can gain information that is useful for evaluating compliance with convention obligations.[50] At the Third Review Conference in 1991, the list of CBMs was expanded to include exchange of data on research centers and high-containment laboratories; declarations on vaccine production facilities; exchange of information on unusual infectious disease outbreaks; encouragement of publication of experiment results; promotion of scientific contacts through international conferences and other fora for exchange; and declaration of legislation, regulations, and other BWC implementation measures. Most important for the purposes here, the CBMs also include "exchange of information on national biological defence research and development (R&D) programs."[51] All BWC member states are encouraged to annually submit to the BWC Implementation Support Unit in Geneva (part of the UN Office for Disarmament Affairs) completed CBM forms covering the previous calendar year. On the whole, however, the annual CBM returns have been few in number. Only 69 states (of the 173 BWC member states, or about 40 percent) participated in the process in 2015 (up from 19 in 1987), and the rate of CBM reporting has exceeded 50 percent only once (in 1991).[52] For some states, nonparticipation in the CBM process might be the result of technical difficulties or a lack of resources and personnel to complete the paperwork. Alternatively, in withholding all or some information, states might simply be eschewing transparency.

In the case of the United States there was no mention of Project Clear Vision or Project Jefferson in its CBM declarations before those projects were revealed by journalists in 2001.[53] Later that year, at the Fifth Review Conference, a senior Chinese official demonstrated his government's sensitivity to what it regarded as hypocrisy in Western demands of developing countries to be more open about their biotechnology activities. He criticized those states that lecture others on BWC obligations while remaining silent about their own relevant activities, remarking, "This is like a man with a flashlight in hand only to cast light on others while he himself stays in the dark."[54] Subsequently, and especially since the end of George W. Bush's presidency, the US government has indicated a growing willingness to be more open about its biodefense program. In 2009, for example, it published a National Strategy for Countering Biological Threats, which stated,

> We will seek to utilize the BWC as our premiere forum for global outreach and coordination on the full scope of risk management activities by . . . [p]romoting confidence in effective BWC implementation and compliance by its States Parties . . . [and] promoting transparency about legitimate activities and pursuing compliance diplomacy to address concerns.[55]

To this end, the US government appears to have tempered its opposition to a BWC verification regime by arranging visits to American biodefense facilities. In late 2009 a senior US official invited Ambassador Pedro Oyarce of Chile to visit the National Interagency Biodefense Campus in Fort Detrick, Maryland.[56] In 2011 the US secretary of state announced a Bio-Transparency and Openness Initiative to commence with "a few state parties to the Convention" being invited to "tour a U.S. biodefense facility."[57] A US official later described the July 2012 tour as one that "achieved . . . our goal to remove misconceptions about ongoing research and showcase that our biodefense work is overwhelmingly open and public."[58]

Such a measure has some potential to alleviate the security dilemma that potentially arises in respect of biodefense activities. Nevertheless, there is room for states to offer reassurance about their peaceful intentions in at least two additional ways. First, individual states could publish (or at least transmit to all BWC member states) the findings of internal, independent reviews. The 2015 CBM report by the United States stated, "The DHS Compliance Review Group, chaired by the DHS Deputy Secretary, reviews all DHS-funded biological defense projects for compliance with the provisions of the Biological Weapons Convention."[59] However, such a review is not independent of government nor is it clear how conclusions about compliance are reached. Canada, by contrast, publishes annual reports by a Biological and Chemical Defense Review Committee composed of three nongovernment scientists. The committee was established in 1990 to assure "the Canadian public, as well as the international community . . . that the Government's policy of maintaining only a defensive capability in this field is fully respected at all times."[60] A second measure that could enhance international confidence in BWC member states' treaty compliance is the declaration of all biological research involving aerosolization. At present, CBM Form A (part 2) requests member states to describe "biological defence work carried out . . . including type(s) of micro-organisms and/or toxins studied, as well as *outdoor* studies of biological aerosols."[61] Laboratory-scale work on aerosols is (by implication) not required to be declared, and yet such work has clear potential for hostile application given that the most efficient way to conduct a mass-casualty biological attack is through the release of an aerosol. This is probably why Germany announced in 2005 that "aerosol experiments" are "avoided in principle" in its biodefense program.[62] As a result of the investigation conducted into the 2001 anthrax attacks in the United States, it became known that US government scientists had for many years been secretly producing lethal *Bacillus anthracis* (Ames strain) bacteria in a readily aerosolized and highly infectious form.[63] This was not, strictly speaking, information that the CBMs required to be disclosed at the time. Nevertheless, it is an activity that arguably warrants disclosure to other BWC member states to assure them that the United States is not leaning toward the weaponization of microorganisms.

Other biodefense activities that bring the "weapon" close to the "biological" might still generate international suspicion and fear, even if information about it were disclosed. In this case, the confidence-building solution would instead be to avoid that activity altogether. Outdoor experimentation with pathogen dispersal mechanisms of the kind conducted by US military scientists at Dugway is a strong candidate for abandonment. This is because such activity, even if it involves only "simulants," brings the United States too close to being in a position to perpetrate biological attacks. A genuine lack of intent to do so is not enough, as the BWC arguably does not allow weapons to be produced even for peaceful purposes. Here, when contemplating the security dilemma, strategic assessment is virtually inseparable from legal judgment; that is, if US activities involving outdoor dispersal systems constitute a breach of Article I of the BWC, then that breach is the strategic equivalent of US "possession" of biological weapons. A high state of readiness to conduct a biological attack would promptly become an object of fear, and this fear could occasion other states to act in ways that risk proliferation.

Under US domestic law, the development, production, stockpiling, transfer, acquisition, retention, or possession of any biological agent, toxin, or delivery system for use as a weapon is prohibited. Significantly, the term "for use as a weapon" is defined to exclude "the development [etc.] . . . of any biological agent, toxin, or *delivery system* for prophylactic, protective or other peaceful purposes" (emphasis added).[64] By contrast, a "peaceful purposes" exception for delivery systems is not available under the BWC, and adherence to the *international* rule is what concerns other states. Article I of the convention prohibits development, production, stockpiling, acquisition, and retention of two categories of object. The first prohibition is on "biological agents . . . of types and in quantities that have no justification for prophylactic, protective or other peaceful purposes" (paragraph 1). The second is on "weapons, equipment or means of delivery designed to use such agents or toxins for hostile purposes or in armed conflict" (paragraph 2). The different treatment of the "biological" versus the "weapon" element is reflected in the different language used. Specifically, whereas a "peaceful purpose" exception exists for biological agents, the BWC categorically bans delivery systems. Such delivery systems are "designed" for a hostile purpose, even if a given state can claim to have a peaceful purpose for working with them; the difference between the words "purpose" and "designed" is critical here. The latter word refers to the engineering features of a physical object rather than the intent of its user. For example, a person might use a rifle for the peaceful *purpose* (at a particular point in time) of testing the strength of bullet-proof vests, but the rifle itself is *designed* (regardless of circumstances) for the "hostile" purpose of firing bullets at people and so killing them.

When commercially available Micronair sprayers and Skil® blowers are operated in the Joint Ambient Breeze Tunnel at Dugway Proving Ground, the US Army is using delivery systems designed for nonhostile purposes. A Micronair atomizer is designed for the agricultural purpose of spraying pesticide on crops, and a Skil® blower is designed for gardening and home maintenance. However, when outdoor delivery systems are used to disperse large quantities of biological simulants toward a target at a particular range (as occurred in 2005), it is a plausible supposition that such systems must have been purpose-built. Although they were used at the time for the peaceful *purpose* of testing biological detection devices, the *design* of the delivery systems must in general have been geared toward generating the threatening effects against which a defense was required. Had the systems not been designed for a hostile purpose and had the "attack" not been realistic, the "threat assessment" rationale for the whole exercise would have been undermined.

An alternative reading of Article I of the BWC is that the "peaceful purpose" exception is incorporated into paragraph 2 by the word "such." In respect of the prohibition on delivery systems, "such agents or toxins" could be read as referring to "microbial or other biological agents, or toxins whatever their origin or method of production, of types and in quantities that have no justification for prophylactic, protective or other peaceful purposes." Outdoor tests involving the dissemination of simulants (nonpathogenic "types" of biological agents) would therefore be justified. However, it is unlikely that this is what the drafters of the BWC intended, and the better interpretation is that "such agents or toxins" refers simply to "microbial or other biological agents, or toxins." In the United Kingdom, which was one of the original depository states for signatures to the BWC, there is no "such" in section 1(1) of the Biological Weapons Act 1974. Instead, the prohibition on delivery systems applies to those "designed to use biological agents or toxins for hostile proposes."[65] The affording of differential treatment to the "biological" and the "weapon" is consistent also with the view of Ambassador James Leonard, the diplomat who led the original US negotiations of the BWC. His explanation for why the language in Article I regarding delivery systems is more restrictive is that the convention was never intended to legitimize the development and production of such systems for defensive purposes. If that *had* been the intention, states would all along have been able to develop and assemble all the technical components necessary for carrying out a biological attack.[66] To allow this would clearly have conflicted with BWC member states' determination, as expressed in the convention's preamble, to exclude completely the possibility of biological agents being used as weapons.

The legal requirement of keeping states removed by one critical step from being in a position to perpetrate biological attacks—the step of weaponization—is, ultimately, one that addresses a strategic concern. To be in that position is dangerous. A state involved in hostilities might, under pressure, resort to the use of an attack capability it had made available to itself, even though attacking other states was not the original purpose behind developing that capability. Were it not for Article I of the BWC—which was deliberately drafted to ban delivery systems categorically—only a change of mind, easily and quickly made, would separate defensive intent from the actuality of offense. Thus, in order to reduce fear and suspicion, and so to alleviate the security dilemma of biodefense, states have a strategic interest in fulfilling a legal obligation: avoid outdoor work with delivery systems that replicate a large-scale biological attack.

CONCLUSION

If a state's biodefense activities are perceived as fearsome, and if fearful states act to reduce their insecurity by engaging in similar activities, there is potential for horizontal proliferation and thus a worsening of the very problem in need of solution. Fear of biological attacks and suspicion of other states' intentions stimulate a security dilemma, and the uncertainty is compounded by the applicability of relevant technologies to purposes benign and malign. Where an offense-defense distinction is able to be drawn in respect to weapons, one state's acquisition of clearly defensive capabilities tends not to be perceived as threatening the security of other states. However, biological weapons do not exist as "weapons" until pathogenic microorganisms are used as weapons. Before that moment, an intention to attack is readily concealed beneath the variety of peaceful purposes to which microbes and associated technologies may be put. Many forms of preparation to defend against future biological attacks are obviously peaceful, but problems of international suspicion are particularly prone to arising when offensive applications of biotechnology are investigated in the name of biodefense. This is the lesson of experience in the United States: certain activities are conducted for "threat assessment" purposes which, if conducted by a rival state, would almost certainly attract

US condemnation. There seems to be a requirement, therefore, for the US government to show greater sensitivity to the role of fear in perpetuating a security dilemma and for other states with biodefense programs to do the same.

In order to reduce the international proliferation pressure resulting from individual states' efforts at self-protection, more states need to exhibit more transparency. For the past four decades the BWC has been underused as a mechanism for reassuring states as to the peaceful purpose behind biodefense efforts. Moving beyond the politically intractable problem of an inspection-driven verification regime, a decrease in the degree of ignorance about states' capabilities would be achieved by greater participation in the CBM process. By revealing and explaining those capabilities to friends and foes alike, individual states would provide general reassurance of peaceful intentions. Uncertainty about intent would remain, but the habit of disclosure would make for a less dangerous condition of uncertainty. Such reassurance would need also to include a commitment to avoid large-scale work with microbe-delivery systems because such activity is both supremely fearsome and probably illegal. When a state places itself in a position to perpetrate biological attacks, ostensibly for the purpose of learning how to organize a defense, the risk is that other states will feel a need to "arm" themselves too. Thereafter, the temptation to attack using this ready capability could one day become difficult to resist. Horizontal proliferation of technical capabilities can thus generate pressure toward use, but so too can proliferation dynamics that are internal to a state. Accordingly, the next chapter extends the discussion of the protect or proliferate dilemma from the international to the domestic sphere, where the potential problem with biodefense is one of vertical proliferation occasioning more threats to a state from within.

NOTES

1. Gregory D. Koblentz, *Living Weapons: Biological Warfare and International Security* (Ithaca, NY: Cornell University Press, 2009), 199.
2. John Herz, *Political Realism and Political Idealism: A Study in Theories and Realities* (Chicago: University of Chicago Press, 1951), 157.
3. John Herz, *International Politics in the Atomic Age* (New York: Columbia University Press, 1959), 241.
4. Ken Booth and Nicholas J. Wheeler, *The Security Dilemma: Fear, Cooperation and Trust in World Politics* (Basingstoke, UK: Palgrave Macmillan, 2008), 9.
5. Robert Jervis, "Cooperation under the Security Dilemma," *World Politics* 30, no. 2 (1978): 187.
6. Ibid., 203–4.
7. Ibid., 204–5.
8. Ibid., 170.
9. Booth and Wheeler, *Security Dilemma*, 1.

10. United Nations Office at Geneva, "Convention on the Prohibition of the Development, Production and Stockpiling of Bacteriological (Biological) and Toxin Weapons and on Their Destruction," April 10, 1972, http://www.unog.ch /80256EDD006B8954/%28httpAssets%29/C4048678A93B6934C1257188004 848D0/$file/BWC-text-English.pdf.

11. Ibid.

12. Filippa Lentzos, "Hard to Prove," *Nonproliferation Review* 18, no. 3 (2011): 572.

13. Ken Alibek, *Biohazard* (London: Arrow, 1999), 234.

14. Jonathan B. Tucker, *Scourge: The Once and Future Threat of Smallpox* (New York: Atlantic Monthly Press, 2001), 145.

15. US Department of State, "2015 Report on Adherence to and Compliance with Arms Control, Nonproliferation, and Disarmament Agreements and Commitments," June 5, 2015, http://www.state.gov/t/avc/rls/rpt/2015/243224.htm.

16. Ibid.

17. Ibid.

18. Booth and Wheeler, *Security Dilemma*, 7.

19. Henry A. Kissinger, "National Security Decision Memorandum (NSDM) 35, United States Policy on Chemical Warfare Program and Bacteriological/Biological Research Program, from National Security Advisory Henry A. Kissinger to the Vice President, the Secretary of State, the Secretary of Defense, etc., November 25, 1969," George Washington University National Security Archive, December 7, 2001, http://www .gwu.edu/~nsarchiv/NSAEBB/NSAEBB58/RNCBW8.pdf.

20. "The Scowcroft Memorandum," *CBW Conventions Bulletin* 57 (2002): 2.

21. Milton Leitenberg, "Distinguishing Offensive from Defensive Biological Weapons Research," *Critical Reviews in Microbiology* 29, no. 3 (2003): 242.

22. Barbara Hatch Rosenberg, "Defending against Biodefence: The Need for Limits," *Disarmament Diplomacy* 69 (February–March 2003): 17.

23. "U.S. Approves Development of Enhanced Anthrax," *Arms Control Today* 31, no. 9 (2001): 26; A. P. Pomerantsev, N. A. Staritsin, Y. V. Mockov, and L. I. Marinin, "Expression of Cereolysine AB Genes in *Bacillus Anthracis* Vaccine Strain Ensures Protection against Experimental Hemolytic Anthrax Infection," *Vaccine* 15, no. 17/18 (1997): 1846–50.

24. Judith Miller, Stephen Engelberg, and William Broad, *Germs: The Ultimate Weapon* (London: Simon & Schuster, 2001), 309.

25. Judith Miller, Stephen Engelberg, and William Broad, "U.S. Germ Warfare Research Pushes Treaty Limits," *New York Times*, September 4, 2001, A1.

26. Miller, Engelberg, and Broad, *Germs*, 295.

27. See Mark Wheelis and Malcolm Dando, "Back to Bioweapons?," *Bulletin of the Atomic Scientists* (January–February 2003): 41–46.

28. George Korch, "Leading Edge of Biodefense: The National Biodefense Analysis and Countermeasures Center," Lecture to the Department of Defense Pest Management Workshop, Jacksonville Naval Air Station, February 9, 2004, Bioweapons and Biodefense Freedom of Information Fund, 2004, http://www.cbwtransparency.org /archive/nbacc.pdf (accessed May 26, 2005).

29. Federation of American Scientists, "Militarily Critical Technologies List (MCTL), Part 2: Weapons of Mass Destruction Technologies, Office of the Under Secretary of

Defense for Acquisition and Technology, February 1998," https://fas.org/irp/threat/mctl98-2/mctl98-2.pdf.

30. Cited in Leitenberg, "Distinguishing Offensive," 235.

31. US Department of Defense, "2014 Department of Defense Chemical and Biological Defense Annual Report to Congress," Chemical and Biological Defense Program, March 2014, http://www.acq.osd.mil/cp/cbd_docs/home/Final%202014%20DoD%20CBDP%20ARC_signed%2021%20Mar%202014.pdfQ1, 9.

32. US Army, "Capabilities Report 2012: West Desert Test Center," Dugway Proving Ground Business Development Branch, 2012, http://www.dugway.army.mil/Documents/2012_Capabilities_Report.pdf, 42.

33. Ibid., 44.

34. United States of America, "Confidence Building Measure Return Covering 2013, Convention on the Prohibition of the Development, Production and Stockpiling of Bacteriological (Biological) and Toxin Weapons and on their Destruction, Submitted to the United Nations on April 15, 2014," United Nations Office at Geneva, http://www.unog.ch/80256EDD006B8954/%28httpAssets%29/7B8EB5C27800D7A9C1257CC3005010BE/$file/BWC_CBM_2014_UnitedStates_PUBLIC.pdf, 44.

35. Sylvie Buteau et al., "Joint Biological Standoff Detection System Increment II: Field Demonstration (Technical Memorandum TM 2006-140)," Defense Technical Information Center, US Department of Defense, December 2007, http://www.dtic.mil/dtic/tr/fulltext/u2/a479297.pdf (accessed July 15, 2014), 11.

36. Ibid., 37–40.

37. US Department of State, "Adherence to and Compliance with Arms Control, Nonproliferation, and Disarmament Agreements and Commitments," August 30, 2005, http://www.state.gov/t/avc/rls/rpt/51977.htm.

38. John J. Mearsheimer, *The Tragedy of Great Power Politics* (New York: Norton, 2001), 45.

39. Shiping Tang, "Fear in International Politics: Two Positions," *International Studies Review* 10 (2008): 453.

40. Commission on the Intelligence Capabilities of the United States Regarding Weapons of Mass Destruction, "Report to the President of the United States" (Washington, DC: Government Printing Office, 2005), 558.

41. Ibid., 501.

42. Yudhijit Bhattacharjee, "Panel Provides Peer Review of Intelligence Research," *Science* 318 (December 7, 2007): 1538.

43. Booth and Wheeler, *Security Dilemma*, 51.

44. "Senate Leader Backs Initiative on Biodefense," *New York Times*, June 2, 2005, A21.

45. Joshua Lederberg, "The Threat of Bioterrorism and the Spread of Infectious Diseases: Hearing before the Committee on Foreign Relations, United States Senate, September 5, 2001," US Government Printing Office, http://www.gpo.gov/fdsys/pkg/CHRG-107shrg75040/html/CHRG-107shrg75040.htm.

46. Donald Mahley, "Statement by the United States to the Ad Hoc Group of Biological Weapons Convention States Parties," US Department of State, July 25, 2001, http://2001-2009.state.gov/t/ac/rls/rm/2001/5497.htm.

47. People's Republic of China, "Statement by H. E. Ambassador FU CONG, Head of the Chinese Delegation, at the 2015 BWC Meeting of Experts

(August 10, 2015, Geneva)," United Nations Office at Geneva, http://www
.unog.ch/80256EDD006B8954/%28httpAssets%29/6E055633A3FB65DEC
1257E9E004FAF06/$file/China.pdf.

48. Nuclear Threat Initiative, "Russia Urges Verification Powers be Added to Bioweap-
ons Treaty Regime," Global Security Newswire, December 8, 2011, http://www
.nti.org/gsn/article/russia-urges-verification-powers-be-added-bioweapons-treaty
-regime/. See also Russian Federation, "Proposal by the Russian Federation for
Inclusion in the Final Document of the Eighth Review Conference of the Biological
Weapons Convention," BWC/MSP/2015/MX/WP.14 (August 12, 2015), United
Nations Office at Geneva, http://www.unog.ch/80256EDD006B8954/%28http
Assets%29/858646FE9CECB76EC1257EA000384422/$file/BWC_MSP_2015
_MX_WP.14.pdf.

49. United Nations Office at Geneva, "The Confidence Building Measures (CBMs),"
n.d., http://www.unog.ch/bwc/cbms.

50. US Department of State, "Hillary Rodham Clinton Remarks at the Seventh Biological and Toxin Weapons Convention Review Conference," December 7, 2011, http://
www.state.gov/secretary/20092013clinton/rm/2011/12/178409.htm.

51. United Nations Office at Geneva, "Confidence Building Measures."

52. Ibid.

53. Jonathan B. Tucker, "Biological Threat Assessment: Is the Cure Worse Than the Disease?," Arms Control Today 34 (2004): 17.

54. Permanent Mission of the People's Republic of China, "Statement by Ambassador
SHA Zukang, Head of the Chinese Delegation, at the 5th Review Conference of the
States Parties to the Convention on the Prohibition of the Development, Production
and Stockpiling of Bacteriological (Biological) and Toxin Weapons and on Their
Destruction (November 19, 2001, Geneva)," United Nations Office at Geneva,
April 16, 2004, http://www.china-un.ch/eng/cjjk/cjda/cj2001/t85217.htm.

55. National Security Council, "National Strategy for Countering Biological Threats,"
the White House, November 2009, https://www.whitehouse.gov/sites/default/files
/National_Strategy_for_Countering_BioThreats.pdf, 19.

56. Ellen O. Tauscher, "Address to the Annual Meeting of the States Parties to the Biological Weapons Convention," US Mission to Geneva, December 9, 2009, https://
geneva.usmission.gov/2009/12/09/tauscher-bwc?.

57. US Department of State, "Hillary Clinton Remarks."

58. Greg Delawie, "Building Partnerships for Biological Threats Prevention, Preparedness and Response," US Department of State, September 5, 2012, http://www.state
.gov/t/avc/rls/197379.htm.

59. United States of America, "Confidence Building Measure Return covering 2014,
Convention on the Prohibition of the Development, Production and Stockpiling
of Bacteriological (Biological) and Toxin Weapons and on their Destruction, Submitted to the United Nations on April 15, 2015," United Nations Office at Geneva,
http://www.unog.ch/80256EDD006B8954/%28httpAssets%29/4631533639F
1D34AC1257E380046511B/$file/BWC_CBM_2015_USA_Public.pdf, 30.

60. Pierre G. Potvin, Julia M. Foght, and Sheldon H. Roth, "2013 Annual Report of
the Biological and Chemical Defence Review Committee," Biological and Chemical Defence Review Committee, December 2013, http://www.bcdrc.ca/CMFiles
/Annual_Reports/English/ar-ra-2013-eng.pdf, 1.

61. United Nations Office at Geneva, "Confidence Building Measures."
62. Germany, "German Policies for Biodefence Research" (BWC/MSP/2005/MX/ WP.10, June 13, 2005), United Nations Office at Geneva, http://www.opbw.org /new_process/mx2005/bwc_msp.2005_mx_wp10_E.pdf, 2–3.
63. Rosenberg, "Defending against Biodefence."
64. United States Code, Title 18, Part I, Chapter 10, section 175, US Government Printing Office, 2011, http://www.gpo.gov/fdsys/pkg/USCODE-2011-title18 /html/USCODE-2011-title18-partI-chap10-sec175.htm.
65. "Biological Weapons Act 1974, Section 1," legislation.gov.uk, http://www.legislation .gov.uk/ukpga/1974/6/section/1.
66. David Ruppe, "Proposed U.S. Biological Research Could Challenge Treaty Restrictions, Experts Charge," Global Security Newswire, June 30, 2004, http://www.nti .org/gsn/article/proposed-us-biological-research-could-challenge-treaty-restrictions -experts-charge/.

2

VERTICAL PROLIFERATION AND THREATS FROM WITHIN

US EXPERIENCE SUGGESTS that some biodefense activities can cause international suspicion and proliferation pressure, but protect or proliferate is a biosecurity dilemma that can arise at the national level as well. Even when state-sponsored research involving pathogenic microorganisms has a genuinely defensive purpose, the nature and scale of that research enterprise might generate risks to public health and national security of internal origin. Since 2001, US laboratory-based research on infectious diseases that could cause biological weapons concern has boomed. More public funds, more laboratory space, and more researchers are now dedicated to biodefense than ever before, and the degree of US effort and expenditure appears vastly to exceed that of any other country. This vertical (internal) proliferation of technical capacity promises increased health benefits in the form of more and better research-based solutions for preventing and treating infectious diseases. Whether a given infection is of natural origin or the result of a biological attack, greater knowledge of the properties of disease-causing microorganisms can lead to the application of more effective countermeasures. Nevertheless, as this chapter will show, there are at least two kinds of risk associated with a research enterprise that involves widely and rapidly "dispersing . . . lethal pathogens throughout the nation."[1]

The first risk associated with the US biodefense boom is that an infectious disease outbreak might be caused by an accident within, or a microorganism's escape from, one of the many US laboratories where research on the most hazardous of pathogens is conducted. The second risk is that, with so many more scientists having access to and knowledge of these pathogens, one or more of those scientists might decide to apply their expertise to the perpetration of a biological attack. If these risks outweigh the aforementioned benefits, the enterprise of biodefense could have the perverse effect of reducing rather than enhancing US security.

THE BIODEFENSE BOOM

Since 2001 the US government has increased enormously its spending on a bio-defense program that involves multiple federal agencies, universities, and commercial enterprises in research and development activities. This increase is mainly a response to the anthrax envelope attacks that occurred in the United States in September and October of that year (causing five deaths), but it is driven also by a concern to protect the American population against emergent infectious disease risks more generally. According to analyses conducted annually at the Center for Health Security (formerly the Center for Biosecurity) at the University of Pittsburgh Medical Center (UPMC), total federal funding for civilian (that is, nonmilitary) biodefense rose from $569 million in FY2001 to over $4 billion in FY2002.[2] This huge and sudden increase in the amount of funding available for biodefense-related research was soon reflected in the awarding of National Institutes of Health (NIH) grants. The number of grants for projects involving anthrax, for example, rose from 28 in 2000 to 253 in 2003. And whereas, in 2000, 25 projects mentioned "bioterrorism" and related words, there were 665 such projects in 2003.[3]

From 2004 to 2009 the UPMC's annual analyses were titled "Billions for Biodefense," but in the subsequent four years they had the more sober title "Federal Agency Biodefense Funding." The last of these (published in 2013) reported that the budgeted amount for FY2014 was nearly $6.7 billion, bringing the total allocation over a fourteen-year period to almost $79 billion.[4] As of 2014, the UPMC no longer provides "a representation of the federal biodefense enterprise" and instead reports on "US government funding for health security."[5] The latter term is defined by the US Department of Health and Human Services as "a state in which a nation and its people are prepared for, protected from, and resilient in the face of health threats."[6] Proposed federal funding for "health security" in FY2015 was reportedly $12.5 billion, but this figure covered budget allocations for a wide range of civilian programs "in biological, radiological and nuclear, chemical, pandemic influenza and emerging infectious disease, and multiple-hazard and preparedness areas."[7] This change in language and scope of analysis obscured what was probably a reduction in government spending for what was once called "the federal biodefense enterprise." Nevertheless, that enterprise today remains a large and expensive one, and the best indicator of this is the amount of laboratory space and personnel dedicated to pathogen research in the United States.

The expansion of US technical capacity for biodefense makes a lot of sense to those who argue that the 2001 anthrax attacks exposed a national shortage: too few of the high-containment laboratory spaces needed to conduct research on microorganisms and develop effective medical countermeasures.[8] Laboratories are characterized as "high-containment" if they are either Biosafety Level 3 (BSL-3) or Biosafety Level 4 (BSL-4) facilities. According to national and international biosafety guidelines, BSL-3 conditions are suitable for work with infectious organisms that may cause serious or lethal disease as a result of exposure by inhalation but against which vaccines or therapies are available. BSL-4 laboratories are required for work with organisms that pose a high risk of life-threatening disease, that may be transmitted by aerosol, and for which there is no vaccine or drug treatment.[9] Until 1990 there were only two BSL-4 facilities in the United States: one at USAMRIID in Maryland and the other at CDC headquarters in Georgia. By 2000 three new BSL-4 laboratories had been built: at Georgia State University, at the University of Texas Medical Branch, and at the Southwest Foundation for Biomedical Research (a privately funded laboratory in San Antonio, Texas).[10] The post-2001 increase in federal funding for biodefense research led to further expansion, and at the time of writing there were thirteen operational or planned BSL-4 laboratories inside the United States.[11] The exact number of BSL-3 laboratories (operated by universities, private corporations, and government agencies) is unknown, even to the US government (which maintains a register).[12] Even so, a 2005 report by the departments of Homeland Security and Health and Human Services estimated that there were then more than six hundred in existence.[13]

All BSL-4 facilities inside the United States are registered with the CDC, which allows them the authority to possess, handle, and transfer so-called select agents (pathogens of bioterrorism concern), and it is probable that most (but not all) US BSL-3 laboratories are CDC-registered too. Official figures on select agent registrations indicate that research in BSL-3 conditions has been the biggest area of expansion in US technical capacity. According to the Government Accountability Office (GAO), there were 415 BSL-3 laboratories registered in 2004, and this number had grown to 1,362 by 2008.[14] During this period the largest increase occurred in the academic sector (from 120 to 474 laboratories), followed by the federal government (from 130 to 395 laboratories).[15] In 2004, 8,335 individuals had CDC approval to access select agents; this number had increased to 10,365 by 2008. Again, the largest growth was in university settings: "In 2004, 2,309 individuals in the academic sector had access approvals; this number increased to 3,110 by 2008 (an increase of 801 workers)."[16] By 2007 the GAO was advising Congress that a "major proliferation of high-containment BSL-3 and BSL-4 labs is taking place in the United States."[17] By 2009 it was estimated that over 15,000 personnel in nearly 1,500 laboratories had authorization to work with one or more select agents.[18]

The important advantage derived from all this additional technical capacity (human resources and physical infrastructure) is that it furthers the US government's biosecurity objective of developing medical countermeasures against infectious disease risks, including biological attacks. According to the National Institute of Allergy and Infectious Diseases (NIAID), scientific research under high-containment conditions on dangerous pathogens and the mechanisms by which they cause disease underpins America's ability to combat infectious diseases. Specifically, such research is considered essential to the development of new and improved diagnostics, treatments, and preventive measures.[19] In 2003, when Boston University and the University of Texas were each awarded government grants of $120 million to build BSL-4 laboratories, Health and Human Services secretary Tommy Thompson described this as "a major step towards being able to provide Americans with effective therapies, vaccines and diagnostics for diseases caused by agents of bioterror as well as for naturally occurring emerging infections."[20] Nevertheless, despite the enthusiasm of government, universities, and corporations for expanding high-containment laboratory space, the vertical proliferation of US biodefense research capacity has sometimes encountered fierce local opposition. In California, Montana, Georgia, North Carolina, New York, Maryland, and Massachusetts, opponents of BSL-4 laboratories have through legal action successfully delayed or prevented the establishment of government-approved facilities and associated research projects.[21] Members of the public have raised concerns that biological weapons will be developed in proposed laboratories, that deadly diseases will leak out because of an accident or a loss-of-containment incident, and that the laboratory and areas nearby would become a target for terrorism.[22]

Regarding the alleged risk of biological weapons development, the problem is not simply that the US government might one day decide to undertake pathogen research for offensive purposes. Rather, it is arguably a cause for concern that, by constantly endeavoring to anticipate threats, the government might be engaged in a dangerous arms race with itself. In the pursuit of "biological security," for example, "biodefense experts" at the Department of Homeland Security's National Biological Threat Characterization Center conduct "studies and laboratory experiments, filling in information gaps to help us better understand and counteract current and *future* biological threats" (emphasis added).[23] In practice this can involve turning "future" (nonexistent) threats into real and present ones, ostensibly in order to devise appropriate countermeasures. A precedent for what could be described as internal arms racing is the US government's development, from the late 1950s to the mid-1970s, of ICBM reentry vehicles (warheads) and antiballistic missile systems. The technical question driving these developments was, Could the former (offense) defeat the latter (defense)? The US government's "intelligence" about its own offensive and defensive achievements informed and inspired efforts to out-achieve itself. As a result, for better or for worse, the rate of technological development was greater than what it might have been had the government sought only to stay ahead of what it thought other national governments were doing.[24]

Reflecting on more recent activities, Melinda Cooper has argued that "the US's sudden [post-2001] preoccupation with bio-warfare needs to be understood, above all, as an effect of the deliberate self-transformation of US defence, a revolution in military affairs that . . . threatens to blur the difference between real and imagined threat."[25] In her view of "the biological turn" in the War on Terror, US activity is mobilized in accordance with the doctrine of preemptive warfare: "The only way to survive the future is to become immersed in its conditions of emergence, to the point of actualizing it ourselves."[26] The implication is that by preempting a biological threat and thereby becoming its originator, the government generates danger (including to itself) where previously there was none. If so, the production for biodefense purposes of genetically novel pathogens is of particular concern. Were such pathogens to escape from the government's control, thus realizing once-imagined risks, the impetus to engage in biodefense research could be regarded as having been a "self-fulfilling prophecy."[27] For example, if scientists created a new and newly dangerous form of influenza virus in order to anticipate the virus's possible natural mutation into that form, they would also be creating (not just researching) a risk to human health. Such an organism, if it somehow escaped from the laboratory in which it was created, would have the potential to sicken and kill many people as it spread. The biosecurity dilemma potentially arising from attempts to regulate research involving novel pathogens is discussed in part II ("secure or stifle"). For present purposes, however, there is ample scope to consider the benefits and risks of wide-scale research on pathogens that already exist.

LABORATORY ACCIDENTS AND UNCONTAINED GERMS

In 1977 a strain of H1N1 influenza, which had disappeared from circulation twenty years earlier, reemerged in human populations in the Soviet Union, Hong Kong, and northeast China. The virus was found to be closely genetically related to a 1950 strain but dissimilar to strains from 1957, suggesting that the new strain had been preserved since 1950. A plausible explanation for the appearance of an "old" influenza virus in 1977 is that it had escaped from a laboratory in which it had been stored.[28] The outbreak of influenza that followed became known as "Russian" flu, even though the first cases reportedly occurred in China.[29] The exact location of the virus's reemergence remains unknown. There is less uncertainty, however, about another disease outbreak of accidental origin that occurred two years later. This outbreak was caused by extensive human exposure to a pathogen inside the Soviet Union, and the pathogen in question escaped from a facility that was probably involved in Soviet preparations for biological warfare. In 1994 *Science* published the findings of an international group of scientists who examined epidemiological data on a 1979 outbreak of inhalation anthrax that had occurred in the city of Sverdlovsk in western Siberia. At least seventy-seven cases and sixty-six deaths were reported, making it the largest such outbreak ever documented. The scientists' conclusion was that, following a failure to activate air filters at a "military facility," the escape and downwind spread of "an aerosol of anthrax pathogen" caused the outbreak.[30] In its effects on public health, this anthrax accident resembled an anthrax attack. The Soviet government presumably harbored no intention to use biological weapons against its own people, and yet Soviet work with lethal pathogens demonstrably posed a public health risk to the extent that it was not conducted safely.

The problem at Sverdlovsk was one of "biosafety," a term that refers to both measures and procedures for protecting the health and safety of people working in laboratories and preventing the accidental release of pathogenic microorganisms into the environment. Physical biosafety measures are barriers or filters between a pathogen and the researcher and between the laboratory and the outside world. The nature of the pathogen being researched (i.e., its infectivity, transmissibility, host range, virulence, susceptibility to vaccination and treatment, and so on) determines the biosafety conditions to be applied. To illustrate, consider the features of a BSL-4 laboratory at the CDC in Atlanta, inside which the *variola major* (smallpox) virus is stored. This lab is supposed to afford conditions of "maximum" containment. The ventilation system there is designed to channel air toward the center of the laboratory, then up and out through highly efficient air filters in the ceiling. If a containment breach were to occur, virus-contaminated air would be retained inside the laboratory through negative atmospheric pressure and not allowed to escape outside and into the surrounding city. For decontamination purposes, all exposed surfaces are bathed in ultraviolet light, which kills viruses. In an anteroom outside the laboratory, scientists entering must remove their street clothes, don surgical gowns and gloves, and climb into blue plastic suits. Each suit has bright yellow rubber gloves securely taped at the wrists, a clear visor hood, and an air valve with a filter protruding from the side. The scientists enter and exit the laboratory through an air lock. When leaving the laboratory, each researcher stands for four minutes under a disinfectant shower to kill any virus particles clinging to the outside of the plastic suit.[31] Preventing the infection of laboratory workers is critical because, if undetected and untreated, such an infection could spread to people in the general community if the pathogen is contagious. In addition, the safe functioning of high-containment laboratories is critically dependent on continuity of electricity supply because electric fans generate the negative pressure that causes air to flow into rather than out of a facility. Preventing the escape of a pathogen also requires crack-free walls, leak-free pipes, and properly sealed doors. If a pathogen were to escape from the laboratory, it might subsequently be spread further by natural forces such as wind, water, or insect-animal vectors. If the pathogen were then to reproduce and establish itself in some niche in the ecosystem, it might for a long period remain a risk to public health.

Laboratory accidents and failures of containment have occurred in the United States even in settings where the strictest biosafety standards are observed, although none of these has proved to be the cause of a widespread disease outbreak. However, the great and rapid expansion of high-containment laboratory capacity since 2001 has undoubtedly increased the probability of accidental infections and noncontainment incidents. The GAO's advice to Congress in 2007 was simple: "There is a baseline risk associated with any high-containment lab, attributable to human errors. With this expansion, the risk will increase."[32] The exact magnitude of that increased risk is difficult to determine, and it might not be proportionate to the increase in the number of people now engaged in pathogen research. But if that risk outweighs the health benefits to be derived from expanding biodefense research capacity, such expansion is counterproductive. For present purposes it is not necessary to describe every reported laboratory accident and biosafety breach that has occurred in the United States during the post-2001 biodefense boom. Rather, it suffices to recall only a select few in order to illustrate the kinds of risks that attend pathogen research in high-containment laboratories.

A good starting point is the initial laboratory-based effort to respond to the anthrax envelope attacks of late 2001 and other numerous "white powder" incidents shortly thereafter. For a period of eight months immediately following the attacks, USAMRIID researchers ran tests on thirty thousand suspicious envelopes, packages, and other items arriving at their facility in Fort Detrick, Maryland. The BSL-3 laboratory that handled *Bacillus anthracis* bacteria normally had a staff of six, but this number swelled to eighty-five to cope with the workload. Many workers learned about handling anthrax bacteria as they worked, and dozens of researchers slept in cars and cots while the laboratory hurried to deal with the flood of specimens. It was a situation in which mistakes and unsafe shortcuts were likely to occur, and in April the following year a researcher detected anthrax contamination outside the institute's laboratories. The discovery caused alarm for three reasons: non-laboratory workers, who were not always vaccinated against anthrax, might have been exposed; anthrax bacteria might have escaped into the nearby town of Frederick, Maryland, when laboratory staff sent away dirty laundry to be cleaned; and someone with access to a contaminated area, and with ill intentions, might have taken away samples of the bacteria.[33]

Later, elsewhere in the United States, a series of safety and containment problems were reported at other laboratories. Some of these were associated with the electricity supply that maintains negative pressure inside research facilities. In 2002, for example, the Plum Island Animal Disease Center in New York experienced a three-hour power outage during a period when replacement workers were filling in for regular workers on strike.[34] In 2005 Hurricane Rita narrowly missed the island of Galveston, where the University of Texas Medical Branch has BSL-3 and BSL-4 laboratories. In preparation for possible physical damage to the labs, and as a precaution against any resulting environmental contamination, Texas researchers shut down their experiments, destroyed research mice, fumigated the laboratories, and locked pathogen samples into freezers plugged into backup generators.[35] In 2007 at a CDC laboratory in Atlanta a grounding cable buried outside the building was cut by construction workers digging at an adjacent site, and subsequent lightning strikes caused a loss of power to the laboratory when the building's circuit breakers disengaged.[36] The following year, another Atlanta-based CDC laboratory was deprived of electricity for one hour when a bird flew into a power transformer. Because no backup generators were operational at the time, the negative air pressure system designed to contain biological agents inside the building shut down.[37]

More commonly, biosafety problems have been associated with human error. For example, in March 2004 scientists at the Southern Research Institute in Maryland sent what they thought were dead *Bacillus anthracis* bacteria to anthrax vaccine research collaborators at the Children's Hospital Oakland Research Institute in California. After tests on mice revealed that the bacteria were in fact live, five Oakland laboratory workers who had been exposed were placed on antibiotics. The bacteria, of the Ames strain, were the same type used in the anthrax envelope attacks of 2001.[38] A similar error occurred soon afterward, but it was more serious because it involved a pathogen that is, unlike *Bacillus anthracis*, human-to-human transmissible. Between October 2004 and February 2005 the College of American Pathologists (CAP) sent influenza testing kits to about thirty-seven hundred laboratories around the world. CAP is a professional organization that helps pathology laboratories improve the accuracy of their testing by sending them mystery samples of various pathogens to identify. On this occasion it had requested a private company—Meridian Bioscience, Inc., of Cincinnati, Ohio—to choose an influenza virus and prepare the test kits. From its stockpile of hundreds of influenza virus strains Meridian managed somehow to select the H2N2 strain, the cause of the 1957 "Asian flu" pandemic that killed an estimated one million people worldwide. Canada's National Microbiology Lab in Winnipeg correctly identified the strain on March 26, 2005, realized its significance, and alerted the World Health Organization (WHO). Because it was generally understood that CAP test kits do not normally carry lethal pathogens, the kits were not handled according to high-level safety standards.[39] As such, there was a risk that a laboratory worker handling the sample might have become infected, potentially resulting in severe illness and the spread of disease to others. Anyone born after 1968, the year the 1957 strain ceased to be included in annual influenza shots, has no immunity to H2N2. To avert the possibility of a laboratory-acquired infection sparking an influenza pandemic, the WHO urged the thousands of scientists who had received vials of the 1957 strain to destroy them immediately. By June 2005 the CDC had announced that all samples had been accounted for and destroyed, and there were no reports of illness.[40]

In January 2005 Boston University revealed that three of its researchers in a BSL-2 (low-containment) laboratory had become ill the previous year after accidental exposure to potentially lethal tularemia bacteria. The exposure had occurred because the researchers had not followed safety procedures requiring them to work with *Francisella tularensis* inside an enclosed box fitted with air filters.[41] In 2006, at Texas A&M University, while cleaning an aerosol chamber a laboratory worker was accidently exposed to bacteria that cause brucellosis. At the time of this incident the worker had no familiarity with the specifics of working with *Brucella* bacteria, and the university lacked the necessary government authorization to be aerosolizing this particular organism.[42] The following year, when it was reported that Texas A&M had failed to report three earlier cases of individuals being exposed to *Coxiella burnetii* (Q fever), the CDC suspended pathogen research at five of the university's laboratories.[43] By this stage the US government was becoming increasingly interested in the kind and number of biosafety incidents occurring at the many high-containment laboratories across the United States. For example, in 2008 the DHS reported that laboratory workers at different sites had accidentally jabbed themselves with needles contaminated by anthrax or West Nile virus and that an air-cleaning system meant to filter dangerous microbes out of a laboratory had failed but no one knew because the failure alarm had been switched off. Other incidents included a batch of West Nile virus, improperly packed in dry ice, having burst open at a Federal Express shipping center, and mice infected with bubonic plague or Q fever having gone missing.[44]

In a 2011 report the CDC identified a total of 395 select agent mishaps (including 196 incidents of "loss of containment") over a six-year period, although the results of a CDC study published the following year painted a picture less bleak.[45] After monitoring over 300 US facilities registered to possess, use, or transfer select agents each year between 2004 and 2010, the CDC study found that (1) there were no reports of theft of any select agent during 2004 to 2010, (2) there was only one instance out of more than 3,400 shipments in which a select agent was actually lost during shipment, (3) there were only 11 laboratory-acquired infections (LAIs) reported to the CDC during the reporting period (1.2 per 10,000 registered workers), (4) there were no fatalities that resulted from any of these infections, and (5) there were no reported cases of secondary transmission to other humans.[46] The key finding was that "the average annual rate of LAIs in . . . facilities registered with CDC was 1.6 per 10,000 authorized workers." Given the higher rate of "occupational illnesses in similar workplaces," the CDC concluded that CDC-registered facilities are "at least as safe, if not safer, than facilities in the overall U.S. research and development sector."[47] Such a rating, while comparably favorable, is nevertheless a poor one. A biosafety accident, unlike a broken leg resulting from a fall at work, has the potential to affect people other than the immediate victim. In particular, if the pathogen concerned is human-to-human transmissible, an accidental, undetected, untreated infection could cause a disease outbreak.

After repeated warnings from the GAO (in 2007, 2009, and 2013) that, "increasing the number of laboratories necessarily increases the aggregate national risk," the moment of political crisis finally came in 2014.[48] Three serious incidents in the US government's own laboratories caused public alarm, after which the government moved swiftly to raise biosafety awareness among scientists. The first involved the potential exposure of scores of CDC employees to live anthrax bacteria after infectious samples were sent to laboratories not equipped to handle them. The second incident involved the contamination of a sample of relatively benign influenza virus (H9N2) with a virulent H5N1 strain. In response to these incidents, health officials imposed a temporary closure of Atlanta-based CDC laboratories engaged in influenza and anthrax research. In announcing the closures, CDC director Thomas Frieden revealed a third alarming incident: the discovery of six vials of *variola major* (smallpox) virus that had been stored in an NIH laboratory since 1954. Two of the vials contained live virus capable of infecting people.[49] The potential exposure of more than eighty workers at three CDC laboratories to the deadly Ames strain of *Bacillus anthracis* appears to have occurred because the bacteria were not successfully inactivated before being shipped to a BSL-2 facility.[50] In the incident involving H5N1 influenza, the cross-contamination of a less dangerous strain of the virus reportedly occurred because a scientist rushed through laboratory procedures in order to get to a staff meeting.[51] As for the vials containing live smallpox virus, these were found in an unguarded storage room.[52]

Frieden declared at a press conference "These are wakeup calls. These are events that tell us we have a problem, and we are going to fix it."[53] And yet, given the US biosafety record of the previous thirteen years, Frieden should not have been "*astonished* that this could have happened here" (emphasis added).[54] Later he told a committee of Congress, "I think we missed a critical pattern. The pattern is an insufficient culture of safety."[55] The 2014 incidents were a "tipping point," Frieden said, that had forced his agency to realize that safety procedures must be improved.[56] Significantly, and consistent with the long-standing advice of the GAO, the CDC director also declared that the number of high-containment laboratories and people with access to dangerous pathogens needed to be reduced to "the absolute minimum necessary"; the greater that number, he reasoned, the greater the risk of accidents.[57] The international dimension of that risk was further illustrated less than a year later when the US Defense Department revealed in May 2015 that a laboratory at Dugway Proving Ground had accidently sent samples of live anthrax bacteria to a number of other laboratories.[58] Those laboratories had been expecting to receive inactive bacteria and, at the time of this writing, the monitoring of individuals potentially exposed to anthrax infection had extended to 194 laboratories in the United States, Australia, Canada, Italy, Germany, Japan, Norway, South Korea, Switzerland, and the United Kingdom.[59]

The proliferation of high-containment laboratories throughout the United States has necessarily been accompanied by an increase in the number of people required to manage those laboratories and conduct research inside them. With regard to the conduct of individuals who handle pathogens, biosafety risk is mainly associated with lack of experience or poor workplace safety culture. Again, the US biodefense boom explains much of the problem. Prior to 2001 the community of scientists who researched obscure diseases like anthrax, Ebola, and plague was a small one. Since then, a great many more researchers have found themselves working on a particular pathogenic microorganism for the first time. The situation is not without precedent; when funding for HIV/AIDS research became available in the 1980s, many scientists poured into this field despite never having previously worked on infectious diseases.[60] But the scientific opportunities presented by the recent biodefense boom have been vast by comparison, and the proportion of relatively inexperienced researchers now working with organisms of bioterrorism concern is high. A 2005 study found, for example, that 97 percent of principal investigators who received NIAID grants from 2001 to 2005 to study six pathogens (anthrax, brucellosis, glanders, plague, melioidosis, or tularemia) were newcomers to such research.[61] The problem of inexperience and the associated risk of accidents is, of course, one that gradually diminishes as individual scientists continue their research. Nevertheless, biosafety risks may persist even in laboratories populated by experienced researchers if the active avoidance of accidents is not a priority.

In university-based laboratories especially, where research tends to be highly dependent on external funding, attendance to biosafety requirements can be unattractively expensive. According to a 2014 estimate, the average cost of training a scientist to work in a BSL-3 or BSL-4 laboratory is $4,000 to $7,000, and training a laboratory administrator can cost around $4,000.[62] There is also the expense of maintaining the high-containment laboratory itself. Universities, glad to receive government funding to plan, design, and construct such a facility, might thereafter find it financially difficult to operate the laboratory safely over time.[63] In large measure, though, biosafety is simply a function of how scientists behave and interact inside a laboratory. After Thomas Frieden appointed Michael Bell to a new position overseeing CDC laboratory safety in 2014, Bell told the *New York Times* that he was most concerned about the "potential for hubris" among researchers who become so accustomed to working with pathogens that they cease to follow safety protocols.[64] Additionally, when an accident does occur, feelings of shame or fear of blame or punishment might prevent self-reporting. When it comes to reporting the mishaps of coworkers and the biosafety failings of supervisors, a scientist might feel constrained by a sense of loyalty, honor, or fear of retribution.[65] Negative publicity, such as that which has surrounded so many of the reported biosafety incidents since 2001, might also be something that scientists seek to actively avoid in order to safeguard future research funding. For all these reasons, and because there are now thousands of scientists engaged in pathogen research, promoting and sustaining a nationwide culture of safety could be difficult. Added to this is the difficultly of preventing scientists from *willfully* endangering other people.

THE SCIENTIST-BIOTERRORIST WITHIN

Beyond the risk of accidents, recent experience in the United States has also highlighted the potential for laboratory scientists to cause harm deliberately. Vertical proliferation of technical capacity for biodefense places dangerous materials and technologies within reach of more individuals, and the associated risk is that one or more scientists might decide to become a bioterrorist. Reasons behind such a decision might include resentment over perceived unfair treatment (such as a reprimand or missed promotion opportunity), financial pressure, blackmail, or psychological or personal problems such as divorce or substance abuse.[66] Whatever the reason, a scientist's desire to cause harm, combined with his or her possession of the microbial means to do so, is dangerous.

In the immediate aftermath of the aircraft-based terrorist attacks of 2001, closely followed as they were by the anthrax envelope attacks, the US government tended to associate the problem of biological "weapons of mass destruction" with external terrorist aggressors. The question that first arose was, Did Al Qaeda, the organization responsible for 9/11, also carry out the subsequent biological attacks? Before long, however, the focus of efforts to identify the likely perpetrator(s) of bioterrorism in 2001 shifted away from the notion of "WMD falling into the hands of (known) terrorists," to the discovery that *Bacillus anthracis* bacteria isolated from the first fatal case of anthrax (in Florida in October 2001) were virtually indistinguishable from bacteria held by the US Army at Fort Detrick.[67] The question then became, Had America been attacked by an American using American anthrax? The idea of a rogue laboratory "insider" was not a new one, and an incident six years earlier provided a glimpse of the dangerous possibility of a biological attack from within. In 1995 a laboratory technician from Arkansas, Larry Wayne Harris, was convicted of fraudulently ordering three vials of *Yersinia pestis* (plague) bacteria from the Maryland-based American Type Culture Collection (ATCC).[68] Harris, falsely representing himself as a microbiologist authorized to receive the bacteria, typed his request on fake letterhead bearing his home address and the identification number of the laboratory where he worked. Fortunately, the suspicions of an ATCC receptionist led to a police tip-off and Harris, a white supremacist and weapons enthusiast, did not obtain any plague bacteria.[69]

In 2001, after anthrax bacteria of US origin was used to cause harm, the scale and intensity of law-enforcement efforts to find the perpetrator(s) was unprecedented. The Federal Bureau of Investigation (FBI) case dubbed "Amerithrax" eventually involved over ten thousand witness interviews, eighty site searches, review of twenty-six thousand emails, analysis of four million megabytes of computer memory, and the issuing of nearly six thousand grand jury subpoenas.[70] Over the course of the investigation the FBI focused on one scientist, Steven Hatfill, who had once worked as a researcher at USAMRIID. The investigators' suspicions proved to be unfounded, however, and Hatfill eventually won a $5.85 million legal settlement when he sued the US attorney general for defaming him as a "person of interest" in the case.[71] Barely a month after Hatfill settled, and at a time when public confidence in the handling of Amerithrax was thus ebbing, the FBI announced that another USAMRIID scientist was the true perpetrator of the 2001 attacks. That scientist, Bruce Ivins, was a microbiologist employed for twenty-eight years by the US Army, and the announcement followed shortly after his death by apparent suicide.[72] This man, if indeed he was acting as a scientist-bioterrorist, was therefore unable to be tried for his alleged crime.

Certainly Ivins knew a great deal about *Bacillus anthracis*. After the 1979 Sverdlovsk outbreak he reportedly abandoned his interest in researching cholera and Legionnaires' disease and turned his attention toward anthrax. After 2001, as scientific interest in the disease boomed, Ivins authored fifteen journal articles, all but one of which focused on possible treatments or vaccines for anthrax exposure.[73] Beyond his publishing achievements, Ivins's work on anthrax vaccines was so well regarded by his employer, the US Defense Department, that in 2003 it awarded him the Decoration of Exceptional Civilian Service.[74] It is unsurprising, then, that the FBI initially called on Ivins (along with other scientists at USAMRIID) to analyze numerous bacteria samples as part of the Amerithrax investigation. Ivins's ability to assist in this way, however, was closely related to his apparent capacity to carry out the anthrax attacks himself. In a 2009 GAO report, that capacity was described in the following terms:

> at the time of the anthrax mailings, Dr. Ivins possessed extensive knowledge of various anthrax production protocols. He was adept at manipulating anthrax production and purification variables to maximize sporulation and improve the quality of anthrax spore preparations. He also understood anthrax aerosolization dosage rates and the importance of purity, consistency, and spore particle size due to his responsibility for providing liquid anthrax spore preparations for animal aerosol challenges. He also had used lyophilizers, biological safety cabinets, incubators, and centrifuges in vaccine research. Such devices are considered essential for the production of the highly purified, powdered anthrax spores used in the fall 2001 mailings.[75]

Furthermore, regarding also the question of his motivation to perpetrate the anthrax attacks, the FBI claimed:

(1) he was the custodian of a large flask of highly purified anthrax spores that possess certain genetic mutations identical to the anthrax used in the attacks;

(2) Ivins has been unable to give investigators an adequate explanation for his late night laboratory work hours around the time of both anthrax mailings;

(3) Ivins has claimed that he was suffering serious mental health issues in the months preceding the attacks, and told a coworker that he had "incredible paranoid, delusional thoughts at times" and feared that he might not be able to control his behavior;

(4) Ivins is believed to have submitted false samples of anthrax from his laboratory to the FBI for forensic analysis in order to mislead investigators;

(5) at the time of the attacks, Ivins was under pressure at work to assist a private company that had lost its FDA [Food and Drug Administration] approval to produce an anthrax vaccine the Army needed for US troops, and which Ivins believed was essential for the anthrax program at USAMRIID; and

(6) Ivins sent an e-mail to a friend a few days before the anthrax attacks warning her that "Bin Laden terrorists for sure have anthrax and sarin gas" and have "just decreed death to all Jews and all Americans," language similar to

the anthrax letters warning "WE HAVE THIS ANTHRAX . . . DEATH TO AMERICA . . . DEATH TO ISRAEL."[76]

The FBI concluded that Ivins was responsible for the anthrax attacks, but the abundant evidence on which it relied was nevertheless circumstantial.[77] No evidence placed him at the mailbox where the anthrax-contaminated envelopes were inserted. As for whether he was solely responsible for the attack, doubt remains regarding the first point in the report because the FBI has not explained how it ruled out as a perpetrator every other scientist who had ever had access to the anthrax flask of which Ivins was the "custodian."

Vahid Majidi, assistant director of the FBI Weapons of Mass Destruction Directorate, admitted to the *Washington Post* in August 2008: "I don't think we're ever going to be able to put the suspicions to bed. There's always going to be a spore on the grassy knoll."[78] Later, the US National Academy of Sciences was commissioned to conduct a scientific review of FBI forensic methods used in the Amerithrax investigation, but the principal finding from the report only stimulated further doubt. The review committee, which was not afforded access to classified information, concluded in its report published in February 2011 that "It is not possible to reach a definitive conclusion about the origins of the *B. anthracis* in the mailings based on the available scientific evidence alone."[79] Despite this finding, a spokesman for the Justice Department told the *New York Times* a few months later "We are confident that we would have proven his [Ivins's] guilt beyond a reasonable doubt at a criminal trial."[80] If Bruce Ivins did not act alone, or if he was framed by the real attacker(s), it follows that one or more scientist-bioterrorists might still be at large. Even if the sole perpetrator of the 2001 anthrax attacks *was* the now-dead Ivins, the broader problem remains: how to reduce the risk of similar behavior by a scientist at any of the many US laboratories where pathogen research goes on. Bacteria that cause the dreaded disease anthrax fall into the category of organisms that can safely be handled in a BSL-3 laboratory. However, as the US government reportedly does not know how many such facilities exist inside the United States, there appears to be no way of accounting for all the places where the preparation of a future biological attack-from-within using anthrax might have (realistically) taken place.

CONCLUSION

The expansion of US technical capacity for biodefense research since 2001— expansion beyond simply the increase of BSL-3 laboratories—constitutes vertical proliferation. Like the horizontal proliferation discussed earlier, it supports but also potentially imperils the goal of protecting populations against infectious disease risks. The benefit of the US biodefense boom has been a concomitant increase in the ability of scientists to research and produce new and better countermeasures against biological attacks and natural disease outbreaks. Yet this vast enterprise of biodefense research has also generated risks of its own. Such is the protect or proliferate biosecurity dilemma that policymakers face in the national sphere. As popular concern about dreaded diseases increases, generating political pressure for more research into defenses against them, there is a simultaneous need to ensure that the technological "solution" does not worsen the problem. With good intentions, but in an uncoordinated rush, multiple US government agencies, universities, and corporations have together increased the number of people and places involved in research on pathogens. That increase has in turn increased the aggregate risk of laboratory accidents resulting in disease outbreaks as well as the risk of bioterrorism originating from within the swollen ranks of capable scientists. Action to reduce those two risks is clearly necessary. However, such action can itself give rise to another kind of biosecurity dilemma: "secure or stifle." How can a government make pathogen research more secure against mishaps and mischief without unduly stifling researchers' pursuit of discoveries that help protect against infectious diseases?

NOTES

1. Michael Baram, "Biotechnological Research on the Most Dangerous Pathogens: Challenges for Risk Governance and Safety Management," *Safety Science* 47 (2009): 892.
2. Crystal Franco, "Billions for Biodefense: Federal Agency Biodefense Funding, FY2009–FY2010," *Biosecurity and Bioterrorism* 7, no. 3 (2009): 292.
3. Scott Shane, "Bioterror Fight May Spawn New Risks," *Baltimore Sun*, June 27, 2004, http://articles.baltimoresun.com/2004-06-27/news/0406270129_1_anthrax -research-biological-agents (accessed June 29, 2004).
4. Tara Kirk Sell and Matthew Watson, "Federal Agency Biodefense Funding, FY2013– FY2014," *Biosecurity and Bioterrorism* 11, no. 3 (2013): 197.
5. Crystal Boddie, Tara Kirk Sell, and Matthew Watson, "Federal Funding for Health Security in FY2015," *Biosecurity and Bioterrorism* 12, no. 4 (2014): 163.
6. US Department of Health and Human Services, "National Health Security Strategy and Implementation Plan," February 13, 2015, http://www.phe.gov/Preparedness /planning/authority/nhss/Pages/strategy.aspx.
7. Boddie, Sell, and Watson, "Federal Funding for Health Security in FY2015," 176.
8. See Nelson Hernandez, "Protesters Decry Fort Detrick Expansion," *Washington Post*, June 6, 2005, http://www.washingtonpost.com/wp-dyn/content /article/2005/06/05/AR2005060501286_pf.html.
9. Centers for Disease Control and Prevention, "Biosafety in Microbiological and Biomedical Laboratories (BMBL), 5th ed.," 2009, http://www.cdc.gov

/biosafety/publications/bmbl5/index.htm; World Health Organization, "Laboratory Biosafety Manual, 3rd ed.," 2004, http://www.who.int/ihr/publications/WHO _CDS_CSR_LYO_2004_11/en/.

10. US Government Accountability Office, "High-Containment Laboratories: National Strategy for Oversight Is Needed," Report No. GAO-09-574 (2009), http://www .gao.gov/new.items/d09574.pdf, 20–21.

11. Virtual Biosecurity Center, "BSL-4 Laboratories in the United States," August 19, 2014, http://www.virtualbiosecuritycenter.org/education-center/us-bsl-laboratories.

12. US Government Accountability Office, "High-Containment Laboratories: Assessment of the Nation's Need Is Missing," Report No. GAO-13-466R (2013), http:// www.gao.gov/assets/660/652308.pdf.

13. Cited in Gigi Kwik Gronvall et al., "High-Containment Biodefense Research Laboratories: Meeting Report and Center Recommendations," *Biosecurity and Bioterrorism* 5, no. 1 (2007): 76.

14. US Government Accountability Office, "High-Containment Laboratories: National Strategy," 24.

15. Ibid., 25.

16. Ibid., 29.

17. Keith Rhodes, "High-Containment Biosafety Laboratories: Preliminary Observations on the Oversight of the Proliferation of BSL-3 and BSL-4 Laboratories in the United States," US Government Accountability Office, Report No. GAO-08-108T (2007), http://www.gao.gov/assets/120/117997.pdf.

18. Frank Gottron and Dana A. Shea, *Oversight of High-Containment Biological Laboratories: Issues for Congress* (Washington, DC: Congressional Research Service, 2009), 3.

19. US Government Accountability Office, "High-Containment Laboratories: National Strategy," 1.

20. National Institutes of Health, "NIAID Funds Construction of Biosafety Laboratories," September 30, 2003, http://www.niaid.nih.gov/newsroom/releases/nblscor rect21.htm (accessed May 10, 2005).

21. Baram, "Biotechnological Research," 896.

22. Kwik Gronvall et al., "High-Containment Biodefense," 82.

23. US Department of Homeland Security, "Biological Security," July 20, 2015, https:// www.dhs.gov/topic/biological-security.

24. Milton Leitenberg, *Assessing the Biological Weapons and Bioterrorism Threat* (Carlisle, PA: Strategic Studies Institute, 2005), 69.

25. Melinda Cooper, "Pre-empting Emergence: The Biological Turn in the War on Terror," *Theory, Culture, and Society* 23, no. 4 (2006): 123.

26. Cooper, "Pre-empting Emergence," 125.

27. Jonathan B. Tucker, "Biological Threat Assessment: Is the Cure Worse than the Disease?," *Arms Control Today*, October 1, 2004, http://www.armscontrol.org/act /2004_10/Tucker.

28. Shanta M. Zimmer and Donald S. Burke, "Historical Perspective—Emergence of Influenza A (H1N1) Viruses," *New England Journal of Medicine* 361 (2009): 282.

29. Edwin D. Kilbourne, "Influenza Pandemics of the Twentieth Century," *Emerging Infectious Diseases* 12, no. 1 (2006): 12.

30. Matthew Meselson et al., "The Sverdlovsk Anthrax Outbreak of 1979," *Science* 266 (November 18, 1994): 1202–8.

31. Jonathan B. Tucker, *Scourge: The Once and Future Threat of Smallpox* (New York: Atlantic Monthly Press, 2001), 224.

32. Rhodes, "High-Containment Biosafety Laboratories," 7.

33. Charles Piller, "Anthrax Leaks Blamed on Lax Safety Habits," *Los Angeles Times*, August 20, 2004, http://articles.latimes.com/2004/aug/20/nation/na-anthrax20 (accessed August 21, 2004); Dan Vergano and Steve Sternberg, "Anthrax Slip-Ups Raise Fears about Planned Biolabs," *USA Today*, October 14, 2004, http://www .usatoday.com/news/nation/2004-10-13-anthrax-labs_x.htm.

34. Marc Santora, "Power Fails for Three Hours at Plum Island Infectious Disease Lab," *New York Times*, December 20, 2002, B10.

35. Jocelyn Kaiser, "Hurricane Rita Spares Major Research Institutions," *Science* 309, no. 5744 (2005): 2143.

36. US Government Accountability Office, "High-Containment Laboratories: National Strategy," 59.

37. Susan Scutti, "The Only Thing Scarier Than Bio-Warfare Is the Antidote," *Newsweek*, March 13, 2014, http://www.newsweek.com/2014/03/21/only-thing-scarier-bio -warfare-antidote-247993.html.

38. Scott Shane, "Live Anthrax Accidentally Shipped from Frederick to California Lab," *Baltimore Sun*, June 11, 2004, http://articles.baltimoresun.com/2004-06-11 /news/0406110389_1_anthrax-bacteria-southern-research-institute (accessed June 14, 2004).

39. Debora MacKenzie, "Pandemic-Causing 'Asian Flu' Accidentally Released," *New Scientist*, April 13, 2005, http://www.newscientist.com/article.ns?id=dn7261 (accessed April 21, 2005); Martin Enserink, "Test Kit Error Is Wake-Up Call for Fifty-Year-Old Foe," *Science* 308 (April 25, 2005): 476.

40. Roxanne Nelson, "Influenza A H2N2 Saga Remains Unexplained," *Lancet Infectious Diseases* 5, no. 6 (2005): 332.

41. Andrew Lawler, "Biodefense Labs: Boston University Under Fire for Pathogen Mishap," *Science* 307, no. 5709 (2005): 501.

42. US Government Accountability Office, "High-Containment Laboratories: National Strategy," 47–49.

43. Jennifer Couzin, "Lapses in Biosafety Spark Concern," *Science* 317 (September 14, 2007): 1487.

44. Denise Grady, "Pathogen Mishaps Rise as Regulators Stay Clear," *New York Times*, July 20, 2014, A1.

45. "CDC Notes Nearly Four Hundred Select Agent Incidents at U.S. Labs," Global Security Newswire, September 29, 2011, http://www.nti.org/gsn/article /cdc-notes-nearly-400-select-agent-incidents-at-us-labs/.

46. Richard D. Henkel, Thomas Miller, and Robbin S. Weyant, "Monitoring Select Agent Theft, Loss, and Release Reports in the United States—2004–2010," *Applied Biosafety* 17, no. 4 (2012): 176–77.

47. Ibid., 179.

48. US Government Accountability Office, "High-Containment Laboratories: Assessment of Nation's Need," 5.

49. Donald G. McNeil Jr., "C.D.C. Shuts Labs After Accidents with Pathogens," *New York Times*, July 12, 2014, A1.

50. Brian Owens, "Anthrax and Smallpox Errors Highlight Gaps in US Biosafety," *Lancet* 384 (July 26, 2014): 294.

51. Lena H. Sun and Brady Dennis, "CDC Scientist Took Shortcuts Handling Deadly Bird Flu Virus, Investigation Finds," *Washington Post*, August 15, 2014, http://www.washingtonpost.com/national/health-science/cdc-scientists-took-shortcuts-handling-deadly-bird-flu-virus-investigation-finds/2014/08/15/893471c8-2403-11e4-86ca-6f03cbd15c1a_story.html.

52. Editorial, "Lapses in the C.D.C.'s Labs," *New York Times*, July 16, 2014, A22.

53. Sara Reardon, "US Disease Agency Suspends Pathogen Shipments," *Nature* (July 11, 2014), http://www.nature.com/news/us-disease-agency-suspends-pathogen-shipments-1.15544?WT.ec_id=NEWS-20140715.

54. Thomas Frieden, quoted in "US Disease Labs 'Made Dangerous Pathogen Transport Errors,'" BBC News, July 12, 2014, http://www.bbc.co.uk/news/world-us-canada-28268640.

55. "U.S. Recovers Hundreds of Misplaced Pathogen Containers," Global Security Newswire, July 17, 2014, http://www.nti.org/gsn/article/us-recovers-hundreds-mis placed-pathogen-containers/.

56. Denise Grady, "C.D.C. Director Admits to Pattern of Unsafe Practices," *New York Times*, July 17, 2014, A16.

57. Grady, "Pathogen Mishaps Rise," A1.

58. Nicky Woolf, "Anthrax Shipment from Pentagon the Result of 'A Massive Institutional Failure,'" *Guardian* (London), July 23, 2015, http://www.theguardian.com/us-news/2015/jul/23/anthrax-shipment-pentagon-institutional-failure.

59. US Department of Defense, "Department of Defense Laboratory Review," September 28, 2015, http://www.defense.gov/News/Special-Reports/DoD-Laboratory-Review.

60. Kwik Gronvall et al., "High-Containment Biodefense," 79.

61. Nick Schwellenbach, "Biodefense: A Plague of Researchers," *Bulletin of the Atomic Scientists* 61, no. 3 (2005): 14–16.

62. Stephanie L. Richards, Victoria C. Pompei, and Alice Anderson, "BSL-3 Laboratory Practices in the United States: Comparison of Select Agent and Non-Select Agent Facilities," *Biosecurity and Bioterrorism* 12, no. 1 (2014): 4.

63. See GAO, "High-Containment Laboratories: National Strategy," 64.

64. Richard Fausset and Donald G. McNeil Jr., "After Lapses, C.D.C. Admits a Lax Culture," *New York Times*, July 14, 2014, A1.

65. Baram, "Biotechnological Research," 893.

66. Jonathan B. Tucker, *Biosecurity: Limiting Terrorist Access to Deadly Pathogens* (Washington, DC: United States Institute of Peace, 2003), 28.

67. "Comparative Genome Sequencing for Discovery of Novel Polymorphisms in *Bacillus Anthracis*," *Science* 296, no. 5575 (2002): 2028–33.

68. Karl Vick, "Plea Bargain Rejected in Bubonic Plague Case," *Washington Post*, April 3, 1996, A8.

69. "Man Arrested in Probe of Illegal Shipment of Plague Bacteria," *Los Angeles Times*, May 17, 1995, http://articles.latimes.com/1995-05-17/news/mn-2852_1_bubonic-plague-bacteria.

70. National Research Council, *Review of the Scientific Approaches Used During the FBI's Investigation of the 2001 Anthrax Letters* (Washington, DC: National Academies Press, 2011), 1.

71. Judith Miller, "Scientist Files Suit over Anthrax Inquiry," *New York Times*, August 27, 2003, A13; Carrie Johnson, "U.S. Settles with Scientist Named in Anthrax Cases," *Washington Post*, June 28, 2008, A01.

72. Carrie Johnson, Carol D. Leonnig, and Del Quentin Wilber, "Scientist Set to Discuss Plea Bargain in Deadly Attacks Commits Suicide," *Washington Post*, August 2, 2008, A01.

73. Sarah Abruzzese and Eric Lipton, "Anthrax Suspect's Death Is Dark End for a Family Man," *New York Times*, August 2, 2008, http://www.nytimes.com/2008/08/02/us/02scientist.html. See, for example, John F. Hewetson, Stephen F. Little, Bruce E. Ivins, Wendy M. Johnson, Phillip R. Pittman, J. Edward Brown, Sarah L. Norris, and Carl J. Nielsen, "An *in Vivo* Passive Protection Assay for the Evaluation of Immunity in AVA-Vaccinated Individuals," *Vaccine* 26, no. 33 (2008): 4262–66.

74. David Willman, "Suspect Stood to Gain from Anthrax Panic," *Los Angeles Times*, August 2, 2008, http://articles.latimes.com/2008/aug/02/nation/na-anthrax2; Amber Dance, "Death Renews Biosecurity Debate," *Nature* 454, no. 7205 (2008): 672.

75. US Government Accountability Office, "High-Containment Laboratories: National Strategy," 38–39.

76. Thomas F. Dellaferra, "Application and Affidavit for Search Warrant Case Number 08-432," US Department of Justice, October 31, 2007, http://www.justice.gov/archive/amerithrax/docs/08-432-m-01.pdf.

77. Carrie Johnson, Del Quentin Wilber, and Dan Eggen, "Evidence Against Scientist Detailed," *Washington Post*, August 7, 2008, A01.

78. Carrie Johnson and Joby Warrick, "FBI Elaborates on Anthrax Case," *Washington Post*, August 19, 2008, A02.

79. National Research Council, *Review of the Scientific Approaches*, 4.

80. Scott Shane, "U.S. Revises Its Response to Lawsuit on Anthrax," *New York Times*, July 20, 2011, A18.

PART II
SECURE OR STIFLE

3

LABORATORY BIOSECURITY

THE BRUCE IVINS AFFAIR awakened the US government to the real and possibly worsening threat posed by trusted laboratory personnel. If a scientist with a high-level security clearance could perpetrate harm against his own country even once, perhaps it could happen again and with consequences more severe. Although US technical capacity to deal with those consequences (using science-based counter-measures) has been enhanced by the biodefense boom, the boom itself has placed a great many more scientists in the type of position Ivins occupied. Whether Ivins was the sole perpetrator of the 2001 anthrax attacks or merely a convenient scapegoat, the length of time it took the FBI to complete its investigation is a factor weighing strongly against the deterrent value of arrest and punishment. Future scientist-bioterrorists might indeed feel confident about getting away with an attack. Beyond deterrence, then, there seems to be a requirement for devising other ways to reduce the risk of biological attacks from occurring in the first place. In 2008, a few months after Ivins's death, the Commission on the Prevention of Weapons of Mass Destruction Proliferation and Terrorism (the "WMD Commission") warned, "The United States should be less concerned that terrorists will become biologists and far more concerned that biologists will become terrorists."[1] When a government decides to act on the latter concern, however, it potentially faces the biosecurity dilemma of "secure or stifle." On the one hand, measures designed to make scientific endeavors more secure can make it less likely that biological materials and related technologies will be instruments of harm to human health. On the other hand, to the extent that security measures stifle the pursuit of lifesaving scientific discoveries, the capacity for research-led protection of human health is undermined.

Laboratory research on pathogenic microorganisms informs clinical and public health measures to protect individuals and populations against infectious diseases. Knowledge of how various bacteria and viruses behave inside the human body enables scientists to develop pharmaceutical countermeasures like antibiotics, antiviral drugs, and vaccines. Alternatively, this knowledge can guide nonpharmaceutical approaches to disease control of the kind discussed in part III of this book. The pursuit of new and better pharmaceuticals tends to be of primary concern, though, and this is increasingly taking place through the application of gene technology. Yet this same technology could in some ways also be applied to the design, development, and use of biological weapons. A scientist who knows what makes a pathogen dangerous (or what genetic mutations could make it more dangerous) is someone who can be regarded simultaneously as a potential source of infectious disease risks and as a valuable ally for governments seeking to resist those risks. Even so, it is not the responsibility of governments alone to govern the behavior of pathogen researchers for the sake of security, science, and public health. These scientists themselves have a role to play, too, and it is in their collective interest to do so.

In this first chapter exploring the secure or stifle dilemma, the focus will be on the conduct of laboratory-based research on pathogenic microorganisms. (The next chapter, on export and publication controls, is concerned with the subsequent dissemination of research findings.) Laboratory biosecurity, which is directly related to biosafety (discussed earlier), involves the "protection, control and accountability for valuable biological materials within laboratories, in order to prevent their unauthorized access, loss, theft, misuse, diversion or intentional release."[2] For the present discussion, it also encompasses regulatory and nonregulatory modes of protection, control, and accountability. That is, laboratory biosecurity is the subject of governance, broadly speaking, and might be based on law or ethics. Whereas the law tends to focus on what may or must be done, ethics is concerned with what should be done. This distinction is important when law-based governance cannot precisely anticipate risks nor balance those risks against the benefits to be derived from research. The first section of this chapter examines the US scheme of laboratory regulation, which is based on a list of biological "select agents" and a requirement that only "reliable" personnel be able to access certain places, materials, and information. The second section discusses the impact of laboratory security rules on the scientific enterprise within and beyond the United States. The chapter concludes with an exploration of some ethical dilemmas arising from pathogen research and the need for a research governance scheme that is integral to the professional status of pathogen researchers worldwide.

SELECT AGENTS AND RELIABLE SCIENTISTS

In the United States, as in many other countries, it is unlawful to develop, produce, stockpile, acquire, or retain biological agents and toxins for a nonpeaceful purpose.[3] Beyond this general prohibition, US law also prescribes detailed rules for the day-to-day activities of individuals with access to certain pathogens. The rules apply to pathogens deemed to be of biological weapons concern ("select agents") and are identified on a published list. Individuals and facilities conducting research on any select agent are required by law to be registered and licensed for that purpose, and enforceable standards govern the secure conduct of that research. Although biosafety regulations have existed in the United States since the late 1960s, biosecurity regulations are relatively new and have been promulgated in three phases.

The first phase began after the 1995 incident in which Larry Wayne Harris fraudulently ordered *Yersinia pestis* (plague) bacteria from a commercial supplier. At the time, the regulation of access to and transfer of biological agents was intended almost exclusively to prevent public distribution of unsafe pharmaceuticals. Thus the only charge on which Harris could be convicted was mail fraud, for misusing a laboratory registration number when placing his order. After this incident, US legislators decided it was too easy to obtain pathogen samples. Under the Antiterrorism and Effective Death Penalty Act of 1996, regulations pertaining to the acquisition, transfer, packaging, labeling, and handling of listed biological select agents and toxins were tightened to reduce the possibility that these could be fraudulently obtained. Henceforth, and with civil and criminal penalties for noncompliance, specific security requirements regarding select agents included facility registration and designation of a responsible official; risk assessments for individuals with access to listed agents; agent transfer rules; safety and security training and inspections; notification after theft, loss, or release of a listed agent; and maintenance of pathogen inventories.[4] At the time of writing, the list of select agents includes sixty-one pathogens that have been determined to have "the potential to pose a severe threat to both human and animal health, to plant health, or to animal and plant products."[5]

The second phase of biosecurity regulation began shortly after the anthrax attacks of late 2001. The USA PATRIOT Act (an acronym for Uniting and Strengthening America by Providing Appropriate Tools Required to Intercept and Obstruct Terrorism) set new requirements for the appropriate use of select agents and specified persons who should be restricted from working with them. The act imposed civil and criminal penalties for inappropriate use.[6] In addition, the Public Health Security and Bioterrorism Preparedness Act of 2002 required laboratory authorities to report all work with select agents and to submit to the Health and Human Services secretary and the US attorney general the names of employees with a legitimate need for access to those pathogens. These names are then checked against criminal, immigration, and national security databases for possible "restricted person" status.[7]

The third and most recent phase of laboratory biosecurity regulation was triggered by the FBI's allegation in 2008 that it was Bruce Ivins who perpetrated the anthrax attacks. In January 2009 President George W. Bush signed Executive Order (EO) 13486, which required a review of the effectiveness of biosecurity policies regarding select agents. The order also established the interdepartmental Working Group on Strengthening the Biosecurity of the United States and was a catalyst for a torrent of reviews and reports by US-based nongovernment organizations.[8] The following year, President Barack Obama's EO 13546 directed the departments of Agriculture and Health and Human Services, as a part of their ongoing biosecurity reviews, to consider reducing the length of the select agent list and establishing higher security standards for select agents with the highest risk of misuse. By October 2012 US biosecurity regulations had been upgraded in respect of thirteen designated "Tier 1" select agents that "present the greatest risk of deliberate misuse with significant potential for mass casualties or devastating effect to the economy, critical infrastructure, or public confidence."[9] Among the Tier 1 agents are those that cause dreaded diseases and are the focus of this book: Ebola virus, *variola major* (smallpox) virus, *Yersinia pestis* (plague) bacteria, and *Bacillus anthracis* (anthrax) bacteria. Other biological agents not in Tier 1 include genetically reconstructed 1918 influenza ("Spanish flu") virus, highly pathogenic strains of avian influenza ("bird flu") virus, and the virus that causes severe acute respiratory syndrome (SARS).[10] The more stringent biosecurity requirements applicable to Tier 1 agents only include, for example, a rule that institutions holding any such agent must have an auxiliary power mechanism (in case of power failure) and have no fewer than three physical security barriers around the area in which the select agent is held.

For the scientists who conduct research on these organisms, the 2012 changes to US biosecurity regulations also included one with direct personal significance: an increase in the frequency of background checks. Individuals granted access to select agents must now undergo a security risk assessment (SRA) every thirty-six months rather than the previous once every five years. The SRA involves an investigation carried out by the FBI to discover any factors that disqualify a person from having access to hazardous materials; disqualifying factors include a criminal history, a substance abuse or mental health problem, a dishonorable discharge from the military, or being a citizen of a state deemed by the US government to be a sponsor of terrorism.[11] According to one FBI official, "the SRA catches people who are dirty already," but beyond that the government is also concerned about security risks associated with people who are vulnerable to becoming "dirty."[12] An individual who passes the SRA might still, for example, be emotionally disturbed or open to extortion to protect embarrassing personal information. For this reason, in 2012 it became a regulatory requirement that organizations in possession of Tier 1 select agents must establish procedures for conducting "pre-access personnel suitability assessments." The idea is that these assessments (performed by the organization itself rather than by a government agency) establish the ability of an individual to comply with biosecurity regulations and also whether he or she displays behaviors that might increase the risk of theft, loss, or release of a select agent. According to the US government, a suitability assessment may include "checking public records for derogatory information, verifying official education transcripts and professional certifications/licenses, and conducting phone or in-person interviews with peer or professional references to obtain additional information."[13]

This official desire to ensure that only suitable (or "reliable") scientists have access to the most dangerous of select agents can be attributed in part to the Bruce Ivins affair and the lesson it provided about the threat of scientist-bioterrorists. Yet the affair itself suggests that participation in a "personnel reliability program" (PRP) might in practice be of dubious value from a security perspective. In 2008, shortly after the FBI publicly accused Ivins of perpetrating the anthrax attacks, a *Washington Post* editorial identified "an urgent need to explain how a man presumably as disturbed as Mr. Ivins was could have maintained a security clearance that allowed him to work with such deadly substances."[14] According to a court-appointed expert panel that later examined Ivins's sealed psychiatric records, Ivins was "psychologically disposed to undertake the [anthrax] mailings; his behavioral history demonstrated his potential for carrying them out." In its 2010 report the panel criticized the USAMRIID managers who had access to Ivins's records for not spotting criminal behaviors and obsessions that he had revealed to mental health professionals.[15] Such information ought to have disqualified Ivins from working with select agents, but he continued to work in his laboratory until November 2007.[16] The fact that the alleged perpetrator of the 2001 anthrax attacks was, at the time and subsequently, the subject of a PRP might be a reason to question the security benefit of such a measure. However, even if the risk of select agent misuse *is* substantially reduced by PRP participation, it is important also to consider the downside, from a biosecurity perspective, of monitoring scientists' reliability.

Prior to the 2012 introduction of personnel suitability assessments, the US National Science Advisory Board for Biosecurity (NSABB) had warned:

> The promulgation of additional [personnel] reliability measures could serve as a powerful disincentive to those who wish to and would responsibly conduct research on select agents because the most talented young researchers, those with many options for research paths, may be far more likely to enter fields with less onerous regulatory requirements. Thus, a burdensome national personnel

reliability program may not only drive scientists from important select agent research, but also drive select agent research out of academia and potentially out of the U.S. into countries with less stringent regulations. Furthermore, the institution of onerous reliability measures could isolate select agent researchers from the mainstream scientific community, isolation that might inhibit research and paradoxically increase the risk of the insider threat.[17]

A few years earlier a report produced by the National Research Council (NRC) had stated, "implementation of the regulatory regime imposed by the PATRIOT and Bioterrorism Response acts on the life sciences community has raised concerns that qualified individuals may be discouraged from conducting biomedical and agricultural research of value to the United States."[18] In essence these were warnings to the US government to navigate carefully the secure or stifle dilemma lest the regulation of research become more injurious than beneficial to public health and national security.

REGULATION AND RESEARCH

Laboratory regulations have clear potential to reduce the likelihood of a scientist using biological materials to cause harm. From a practical perspective alone, material- and personnel-based restrictions raise the difficulty threshold for initiating a biological attack, and this much is good news from a public health perspective. At the same time, however, a health-based argument could be made against any regulatory scheme that scientists perceive to be overly strict. If the burden of biosecurity regulation causes too many scientists to opt out of pathogen research, the result could be a gradual and overall diminution of scientific capacity to understand and manage infectious disease risks. Weighing against this possibility is the existence, particularly in the United States, of a well-funded biodefense industry attracting talent and dispersing grants for research on organisms that people might be exposed to in a biological attack or a natural disease outbreak. Nevertheless, in this context the policy challenge is to maximize scientific opportunities and minimize opportunity costs, even though the latter can be difficult to measure.

Some pathogen researchers might argue that the quantity and quality of their scientific output would be greater but for the abundance of regulations to which they must adhere. At present, institutions that receive government funding are legally required to conduct reviews of research involving animals, human subjects, or recombinant DNA. Individual scientists must adhere to safety-training requirements and must follow ethical guidelines covering intellectual property,

conflicts of interest, and authorship of scientific papers. Thus, even before biosecurity is taken into account, laboratory-based biological science is a regulation-
rich scene. And yet, biosecurity regulations are liable to be regarded as overly or
unnecessarily burdensome, from a scientist's perspective, precisely because the
problem to be avoided (an insider threat) is neither regularly encountered nor
immediately apparent. As five members of the NSABB wrote in 2009, "the regulation of responsible scientists and legitimate technologies and microbes with
the goal of eliminating a threat that may involve 1 individual among 10 million humans is tricky business." They added: "We cannot really know if we've
over-regulated to the detriment of science in the U.S. because it is impossible
to estimate the cost of research that is not done."[19] Since the start of the biodefense boom, the amount of pathogen research that *is* done has increased, but one
problem with US biosecurity regulations might be that they cause such research
to be done less efficiently. In one study of bibliometric data, the results of which
were published in 2010, the analysts hypothesized: "If the counter bioterrorism
laws have had detrimental effects on select agent research, the impacts should be
detectable in the published literature, the output by which scientific production
is judged."[20] Focusing on the literature on *Bacillus anthracis* and Ebola virus, the
study found that the average number of annual publications increased after 2002
but that there was a steep decline in the number of papers per million dollars of
US government funding (a two- to fivefold fall in efficiency) for each select agent.
A key finding was that the average cost of a research paper on the Ebola virus
had increased from about US$59,000 to $333,000 over the period when more
restrictive biosecurity regulations were adopted in 2001 and 2002.[21]

More generally, there is some evidence that biosecurity regulations have had
a chilling effect on pathogen research within the United States, as the burden of
monitoring and reporting has generated a disincentive to work with select agents.
Since 2001 there have been signs of scientists' keenness to escape the reach of
unwelcome regulation. For example, in October of that year, Iowa State University destroyed its entire collection of anthrax samples;[22] later, another two hundred institutions either transferred or destroyed their select agent inventories so
as to avoid the need for registration under new biosecurity legislation.[23] In 2010
two US microbiologists conducted a questionnaire-based survey of one thousand
individuals in "the biosafety community" and received thirteen confirmations
that a collection of microbes had been destroyed in response to regulations governing select agents.[24] Such destruction, which the surveyors suspected was more
extensive than reported, represented "a loss of strains and biological diversity
available for biomedical research."[25] Even so, it seems that at least some US scientists have not regarded the benefit of retaining stocks of select agents as outweighing the burden of associated regulation. Stanford University microbiologist

Stanley Falkow, for example, told the *New York Times* in 2004 "These rules affect not just scientists who work with me, but [also] those who clean labs and all who have access to them. It's just not worth it."[26] The previous year one of Falkow's colleagues, Thomas Butler of Texas Tech University, had been found guilty of violating biosecurity regulations and imprisoned, and some US scientists have cited this as a reason for avoiding work with select agents.[27] Butler had shipped *Yersinia pestis* (plague) samples from Tanzania (where a natural outbreak of the disease was ongoing) to other researchers inside the United States but without adequate labeling of the packages and without a government-issued permit for international transfer.[28] Although his action—sharing his findings about the effectiveness of certain antibiotics against plague infection—could be regarded as essentially protective against an infectious disease, it was judged to carry too great a risk of an accidental or deliberate release of deadly bacteria.[29]

It is difficult to know how or the extent to which Thomas Butler's brush with the law has affected the attitudes and behavior of other US-based pathogen researchers. It might have encouraged some scientists simply to adhere more carefully to biosecurity regulations. But it might also have served as a general disincentive for other scientists to conduct research involving select agents.[30] Regarding the latter possibility, the concern is that this could have repercussions for public health in the sense that lifesaving scientific discoveries might be foregone. Other scientists less concerned by the prospect of becoming "the next Thomas Butler" might nevertheless find that from a purely practical perspective, biosecurity regulations make pathogen research intolerably difficult. This too could be a research disincentive with public health implications, especially if (as is often and increasingly the case) a pathogen subjected to US regulation is being studied collaboratively by an international team of scientists. In 2003 international collaboration had facilitated a rapid strengthening of the scientific basis for responding to the SARS outbreak, with scientists in laboratories in Canada, the United States, the Netherlands, and Germany contributing to the full genetic sequence of the SARS virus. Yet, as Julie Fischer has observed, such speedy collaboration transcending national borders would probably not have been possible had the virus been the subject of biosecurity controls.[31] When the US government listed the SARS virus as a select agent in 2012, the local impact was that thirty-eight US laboratories holding the virus had until April the following year to either upgrade their security measures or destroy or transfer their stocks.[32] To the extent that laboratories opted for the latter, it could be argued that select agent regulations effectively reduced US scientific capacity regarding SARS. The broader impact, however, was that US biosecurity regulations made it more difficult for US scientists to share materials and data with international partners working on the SARS virus (or any select agent, for that matter) in relatively underregulated laboratories abroad. This now presents a problem for foreign scientists, too, because US expertise is often highly valued in countries where a disease caused by a select agent is endemic.

In the circumstance of inconsistent conditions of laboratory biosecurity, only two policy approaches suggest themselves: either to allow non-US scientists to work in US laboratories or to require non-US laboratories to operate in accordance with US security standards. The problem with the first approach is that foreign scientists seeking to conduct research on a select agent in the United States (perhaps because the disease it causes is a serious health burden in their home country) must first be deemed reliable. Passing the SRA or participating in a PRP (in the case of a Tier 1 agent) might, depending on a scientist's country of origin, be more difficult in practice than it would be for a US scientist. This is because the US government has long been concerned that allowing foreigners into US laboratories might increase the risk of pathogen misuse. Since 2001 the PATRIOT Act has prohibited any researcher who hailed from a terrorism-sponsoring country from handling select agents in the United States, regardless of whether he or she has a clean record. In the case of scientists who are not from such countries, establishing their reliability could still be difficult because of differential vetting standards. That is, accepting background checks and personnel security evaluations conducted in foreign countries might not be feasible if, for example, different definitions of the term "adjudicated mental defective" apply to people outside the United States.[33] From a biosecurity perspective it makes sense on the one hand to apply the same reliability checks on US and non-US scientists in order to reduce the risk that anyone with access to a select agent will abuse his or her position to perpetrate a biological attack. On the other hand, non-US scientists might well feel a pressing need to share in the potentially lifesaving discoveries taking place in US laboratories. As an African delegate at a WHO research meeting in Geneva told US journalist Laurie Garrett in 2013,

> We are the ones that actually suffer from all of these diseases. We are the ones that need this research. But we cannot do it. We do not have the facilities. We do not have the resources. And now . . . our people cannot get into your laboratories to work by your side for security reasons.[34]

Even if the health concerns of other countries are set aside, there remains the possibility that US laboratory biosecurity regulations are bad for the United States itself, to the extent that international scientific collaboration is inhibited. In 2006 a committee of the NRC observed, "As technological growth becomes increasingly dependent on the global commons, international scientific exchanges and collaborations become an ever more vital component of U.S. technological capacity, including biodefense technological capacity."[35] The following year, two other

NRC committees stated, "We must . . . remain open to the benefits that foreign-born, but U.S.-trained, scientists and engineers bring to our country in terms of technological and economic growth."[36] In 2009 another recommendation from the NRC came: "The President should maintain and enhance access to the reservoir of human talent from foreign sources to strengthen the U.S. science and technology base."[37] Achieving all this seems to require, among other things, that international collaboration on pathogen research involving US-based scientists remains attractive. Militating against this, however, are the personnel problems associated with internationally inconsistent security standards. Moreover, the second approach to addressing this inconsistency—requiring non-US laboratories to operate in accordance with US standards—is arguably even more problematic.

The science-based argument in favor of globalizing (US) laboratory biosecurity standards tends to be that regulations applicable only within the United States put US scientists at a competitive disadvantage (the biodefense boom notwithstanding).[38] The security-based argument is that strict laboratory rules only shift rather than reduce the global scientist-bioterrorist threat, such that the United States remains vulnerable to threats emanating from unregulated (or underregulated) foreign laboratories.[39] When these two perspectives are combined, a fearsome prospect emerges: an increase in the global threat of biological attacks as non-US laboratory capacity expands alongside a relative decrease in US technical capacity to respond to infectious disease risks. Perhaps this problem would be less severe if more national governments regulated pathogen research as strictly as the US government does. However, in many parts of the world, the fact that the select agents covered by US rules are endemic (and thus abundantly available) means that rules like these are impractical. In addition, given that some poorer countries struggle constantly to manage heavy infectious disease burdens of natural origin, it is likely to be politically unacceptable for governments to invest resources in laboratory biosecurity rather than in outbreak response and healthcare capacity.

Despite such objections to the "globalization" of laboratory biosecurity, it is hard to deny that biological weapons are a potential threat to everyone everywhere and not just to Americans in the United States. Therefore, for the sake of humanity in general, there is a strong case for some kind of risk-reduction effort on a global scale. But that effort need not involve simply expanding the regulatory reach of government into more laboratories in more countries. Even if this were possible it would be inadequate. As the next section shows, many of the risks associated with certain kinds of pathogen research are not wholly susceptible to rigid, top-down modes of governance. Accordingly, governance of that research might need to be "global" in a nongeographical sense: encompassing a diversity of approaches (law based and ethics based) and participants (governments and nongovernment actors).

RESEARCH DILEMMAS AND PROFESSIONAL ETHICS

As the 2001 anthrax attacks demonstrated, the theft and harmful misuse of hazardous pathogens is a risk to public health, and addressing that risk is an important policy challenge. For at least two reasons, however, the registration and attempted control of physical quantities of certain organisms is an inadequate response to the broader potential problem of using biotechnology for destructive purposes. First, in the course of laboratory-based experimentation, risks can arise in situations where registered pathogens are being studied in a highly secure laboratory environment, but they can also arise in connection with research on unregistered nonpathogens that is conducted in workspaces with fewer safeguards in place. Second, access to disease-relevant biotechnology is becoming harder to monitor as, increasingly, that technology is acquired and transferred in an intangible (nonphysical) form. In this context, and with the pace of microbiological science advancing rapidly, traditional forms of governance based on an arms-control model (envisaging the control of physical items) are unlikely to succeed on their own. Rather, reducing the security risks associated with laboratory research seems also to require a governance approach that is more flexible in its application and more comprehensive in its effect on day-to-day scientific practices.

When biological weapons are conceived of as "weapons of mass destruction," an erroneous assumption is sometimes made that hazardous biological substances can be tracked and controlled in a manner similar to that applied to fissile nuclear substances (e.g., plutonium or highly enriched uranium). Since the time of the 2001 anthrax attacks, however, this assumption has gradually been replaced by an awareness that the same approach does not translate well to the biological realm. By 2009, for example, former US senators Bob Graham and Jim Talent (co-chairs of the WMD Commission) were arguing: "Given the vast differences in the weaponization of nuclear and biological technologies, it is important to have a biological weapons prevention strategy that does not merely involve crossing out 'nuclear' and adding 'bio.'"[40] Indeed, on the matter of limiting access to critical materials, there are three important differences when it comes to biological weapons. First, almost all biological agents that endanger human health are found naturally in the environment, and many are stored at countless government, university, and commercial laboratories around the world. Second, in contrast to visible fissile materials that exist in small quantities, pathogenic microorganisms are invisible (microscopic) and so numerous as to be beyond counting. Third, biotechnology advancements are increasingly enabling scientists to chemically synthesize the entire genetic code of microorganisms, thus obviating the need to ship live biological agents in the same way that fissile materials are shipped. As a consequence of these factors, attempts to control physical quantities of certain pathogens by means of biosecurity regulations are clearly insufficient.

A law-based, materials-based regulatory approach to the governance of laboratory-based pathogen research is not an approach that can anticipate the variety of ways in which the fruits of that research could be misapplied. It is also not an approach that explicitly and systematically accounts for the many health benefits that pathogen research can or could achieve. Overwhelmingly the scientists who conduct this research have in mind the benign application of any new technology discovered through laboratory experimentation. Therefore, for governance purposes it is unhelpful and unfair to regard such work only as a source of disease risk. Rather, the balance of likely risks *and* the benefits arising from research need to be contemplated by policymakers and by the scientists themselves. A set of legal regulations cannot provide an answer to the question of whether a particular research activity is *worth* the associated risk, because this is essentially an ethical question that demands the weighing of different and potentially competing values: national security, public health, academic freedom, and so on. Scientists who adhere to biosecurity regulations while conducting research on select agents might still face ethical dilemmas in their work, just as scientists who conduct research on nonlisted pathogens or on nonpathogenic organisms do. That is, when bearing in mind risks and benefits, such scientists might feel doubts about whether a particular line of research should be pursued or how that research should be conducted. A dilemma might also arise on the question of whether or how the findings of pathogen research should be communicated to others, and this is discussed at length in chapter 4. For now, though, it suffices to focus on the actual conduct of research and the need for research governance mechanisms that require scientists to engage professionally with ethical questions as well as with legal rules. It is a need that can be illustrated by some examples of the dual-use dilemma that scientists sometimes encounter in their work.

The Dual-Use Dilemma

Biotechnology, along with virtually all other technologies, has the potential to be used for both benign and malign purposes. This potential for "dual use" rarely poses a policy challenge because in practice the benefit of the widespread application of most technologies for beneficial purposes far outweighs the risk of harmful misuse. Governments do not, for example, regulate the possession and transfer of writing paper (one component of communication technology) on public safety grounds, even though a piece of paper could be ignited and used to start a destructive fire. Dual-use technology is distinguishable, however, from technology that poses a dual-use *dilemma* because the preponderance of benefits over risks associated with its application (or vice versa) is not obvious. In such circumstances, when the populace's health is the object of concern, the policy challenge is to govern access to and use of a particular technology in a way that is likely to achieve more good than harm. Here, "good" includes both actual benefits and avoided harms; "harm" includes both actual harm and forgone benefits.

In the realm of molecular biology, due to advances in gene modification and synthesis techniques, it is now possible to make pathogenic microorganisms (and to make microorganisms pathogenic) in a laboratory setting. Scientists can make use of such technology in order to, among other things, investigate the potential for a microorganism's genome to mutate naturally and so present a new kind of disease risk. By anticipating that risk, the findings of research into the nature and behavior of a genetically mutated microorganism can then inform the preparation of clinical and public health responses. A scientist might, for example, set out deliberately to generate a bacterium resistant to a certain class of antibiotics in order to determine whether it could become resistant to that class through natural processes. Such information would be relevant to recommendations on how best to administer an antibiotic, or it could help guide the medical management of infectious disease cases. Alternatively, however, laboratory work of this kind also can lead to making a pathogen more useful for biological attack purposes precisely *because* that pathogen has been rendered capable of defeating the defenses erected by the human immune system and the supplementary defense afforded by a vaccine or drug. The ethical question then is whether the risks associated with a particular experiment of this kind outweigh the likely benefits. If the answer does not seem obvious, a dual-use dilemma has arisen.

In a report titled *Biotechnology Research in an Age of Terrorism* published by the NRC in 2004, seven kinds of experiments were identified as those most likely to have biological weapons potential: (1) if the experiment could demonstrate how to render a vaccine ineffective, (2) if the experiment could confer resistance to therapeutically useful antibiotics, (3) if the experiment could enhance the virulence of a pathogen or render a nonpathogen virulent, (4) if the experiment could increase the transmissibility of a pathogen, (5) if the experiment could alter the host range of a pathogen, (6) if the experiment could enable the evasion of diagnosis or detection by established methods, and (7) if the experiment could enable the weaponization of a biological agent.[41] More recently, the US government has used the term "dual-use research of concern" (DURC) in relation to a similar list of experiment categories, and it has done so in the context of a policy for reviewing pathogen research (for risk-mitigation purposes) that is government-conducted or government-funded. The policy applies only to fourteen biological agents, most of which are also Tier 1 select agents. It defines DURC as

> life sciences research that, based on current understanding, can be *reasonably* anticipated to provide knowledge, information, products, or technologies that could be *directly* misapplied to pose a significant threat with broad potential consequences to public health and safety, agricultural crops and other plants, animals, the environment, material, or national security (emphasis added).[42]

Inevitably, informed opinions will differ as to what counts as "reasonable" anticipation or a "direct" threat, but in essence the judgment this policy requires of researchers and reviewers is to decide whether the risks associated with a particular experiment outweigh the benefits to be derived. In 2005 such a judgment had to be made with regard to research into what made the 1918 Spanish flu virus so virulent. Using the recently completed genetic code sequence of this virus (obtained from the preserved tissue of long-dead victims), researchers had generated a virus identical to that which caused the worst pandemic of the twentieth century.[43] When this activity was revealed publicly, critics argued that the mere existence of such a virus generated an unacceptable risk, such as accidental release into the human population, the theft and harmful misuse of the virus by a laboratory worker, or a decision by a hostile state to reconstruct its own version of the virus for biological warfare purposes. But the counterargument prevailed: because the scientists' discovery produced knowledge that was useful for improving preparedness for a future influenza pandemic, the public health upside to this research sufficiently outweighed these risks.[44]

A similar justification—of benefits outweighing risks—was later offered by other scientists who produced a different kind of pandemic influenza virus which, unlike Spanish flu, had never appeared in nature. However, the production in 2011 of a new, more transmissible version of the H5N1 bird flu virus generated much more controversy over the dual-use dilemma associated with this research. Two rival teams of influenza researchers—one in the United States and one in the Netherlands—were involved in producing such a virus, and the work of both teams was funded by the NIH. The US team, led by Yoshihiro Kawaoka of the University of Wisconsin–Madison, engineered a virus expressing H5N1 and H1N1 (2009 "swine flu") genes that was capable of airborne spread between ferrets (an animal model chosen for the similarity of its respiratory system to humans').[45] The Dutch team, led by Ron Fouchier of the Erasmus Medical Centre in Rotterdam, used a combination of genetic engineering and serial infection of ferrets to develop a mutant H5N1 virus that could likewise spread among the animals without direct contact.[46] Both sets of experiments were conducted in a high-containment ("BSL-3+") laboratory. Kawaoka's mutant virus did not kill any of the ferrets infected during the course of experimentation, but Fouchier's did. In each case, though, a genetically new and presumably human-to-human transmissible influenza virus had come into existence inside a laboratory. The ethical question that was debated only much later was whether such experimentation should have been done at all. Did the benefits outweigh the risks?

The scientists involved certainly thought so, and so did the NIH, which had for several years been funding similar research by numerous teams aimed at showing how the H5N1 virus might acquire the ability to spread between humans.[47] Adopting a public health perspective, Kawaoka explained in 2012: "Given the potential consequences of a global outbreak, it is crucial to know whether these viruses can ever become transmissible."[48] The knowledge gained from this kind of "gain-of-function" (GoF) experiment might indeed be beneficial if, for example, it could be used to convince policymakers that the risk of a pandemic of H5N1 influenza is real and thus worthy of funding strategies to contain it. Also, in knowing which genetic mutations are needed for increased transmissibility, H5N1 surveillance teams around the world could look out for these mutations in viral samples taken from infected birds and humans. A laboratory-created pandemic virus could also be used to test and perhaps improve the effectiveness of existing influenza vaccines and antiviral drugs. However, there are also good reasons for thinking that the benefit to public health of Kawaoka's and Fouchier's experiments might not be so great. If multiple mutation pathways exist by which H5N1 could achieve human pandemic potential, the genetic characteristics of such a virus that emerges naturally could differ substantially from one created in a laboratory. This in turn could undermine the public health value of conducting any prepandemic testing or the development of pharmaceutical countermeasures. From a disease surveillance perspective, it might be impractical or impossible to detect a specific viral mutation in nature quickly enough to allow an opportunity to stop a virus spreading.

Uncertainty or pessimism about the benefits of GoF experiments may lead to an assessment that the risks thereof are a more weighty concern. High-containment laboratories and "reliable" scientists notwithstanding, an artificial pandemic influenza virus might escape or be stolen and misused. The likelihood of a scientist being infected accidentally, for example, has been calculated as approaching 20 percent over a ten-year period. This was the figure arrived at by Marc Lipsitch and Alison Galvani who, in a 2014 article, presented an ethical argument against what they called "potential pandemic pathogen" (PPP) experiments. According to Lipsitch and Galvani, the H5N1 research by Kawaoka and Fouchier should not have been pursued because, "there are safer experimental approaches that are both more scientifically informative and more straightforward to translate into improved public health through enhanced surveillance, prevention, and treatment of influenza."[49] Other approaches "being pursued without risks of PPP release," they argued, include "developing universal influenza vaccines and novel antiviral drugs and strategies to enhance host responses, as well as improving technologies for rapid vaccine manufacture."[50] In response to their argument, Fouchier insisted that "scientific research has never triggered a virus pandemic."[51] Earlier he had offered the assurance that "if I did infect myself, we [the Erasmus Medical Centre] have isolation wards in the adjacent hospital. . . . It's practically impossible for one of my team members to accidentally take the virus along into the Rotterdam subway."[52] The assumption underlying the latter claim is that an accidental infection would always be detected at the time, but of course undetected infections (such as with the SARS virus) have happened before.[53]

In early 2012 thirty-nine of the world's leading influenza virus researchers (including Fouchier and Kawaoka) demonstrated their sensitivity to public concern when they published a letter committing themselves to a research moratorium. Voluntarily, and for a period that eventually exceeded one year, these scientists eschewed "any research involving highly pathogenic avian influenza H5N1 viruses leading to the generation of viruses that are more transmissible in mammals."[54] Even so, GoF research on influenza viruses resumed in 2013 and the ethical debate intensified. Scientists opposed to such research organized themselves into the Cambridge Working Group (see www.cambridgeworking-group.org), and those in favor issued public statements as Scientists for Science (www.scientistsforscience.org). Then, in 2014, the debate was overtaken by an extraordinary decision by the US government in response to the earlier revelation of a series of biosafety incidents at CDC laboratories (see chapter 2). The White House Office of Science and Technology Policy announced a goal to "promote and enhance the nation's biosafety and biosecurity" and launched a deliberative process to assess the potential risks and benefits associated with GoF experiments; all federal funding for the conduct or encouragement of such research was halted until the process was concluded.[55] Some scientists reacted with dismay that the government was effectively preventing or discouraging potentially lifesaving research.[56]

A research moratorium (whether voluntary or government-imposed) is a drastic and reactive governance mechanism; a better approach would be one in which pathogen researchers were proactive in routinely anticipating and managing dual-use dilemmas. As the next chapter will show, deliberation about the benefits and risks of Fouchier's and Kawaoka's GoF research occurred at a very late stage (when research findings were ready to be disseminated), and there was little consideration of the dual-use implications when these influenza virus projects were proposed, reviewed, and funded. In hindsight it is clear that risks and benefits should have been carefully considered in a more timely fashion. This need can be recognized more generally, not only from a national security or public health perspective but also in terms of the collective interests and responsibilities of pathogen researchers. That is, when it comes to the dual-use dilemma, the governance of pathogen research should be approached as a matter of professional ethics. Such governance should be global in the sense of being "owned and operated" by scientists worldwide, and any universal protocols would supplement rather than replace national-level, law-based mechanisms for regulating laboratory biosecurity.

Ethics-Based Governance

National laws govern the behavior of individuals within a given territory and international laws govern the behavior of states, but law-based governance is difficult to globalize. Inevitably the behavior of some people in some parts of the world will remain beyond the reach of regulation. Moreover, it is often the case that top-down forms of governance are resented and resisted by people who place a high value on individual freedom of action. Scientists in particular exhibit a keenness for the pursuit of knowledge unhindered, and yet it is also the case that science itself is facilitated by conditions of good public health and societal stability. Thus the relationship between science, health, and national security can be perceived and approached from a bottom-up perspective too. With regard to pathogen research and biosecurity, the notion of bidirectional governance has been in political favor among governments for more than a decade. For example, the final report of the 2008 meeting of BWC member states noted "the importance of balancing 'top-down' government or institutional controls with 'bottom-up' oversight by scientific establishments and scientists themselves."[57] To date, however, little of the latter has been forthcoming from pathogen researchers or the organizations that represent them nationally and globally. This might appear at first to be a professional failing on the part of these scientists, except that their collective status *as* a profession is uncertain.

A "professional" is someone who pursues a "higher calling" in the service of society. Among the members of any profession there is generally a sense of corporate unity and a consciousness of the group as set apart from others. This collective identity has its origins, according to Samuel Huntington, "in the lengthy discipline and training necessary for professional competence, the common bond of work, and the sharing of a unique social responsibility."[58] In many parts of the world a professional sense of responsibility to society is evident among, for example, accountants, teachers, engineers, and lawyers. The professionalism of medical practitioners is particularly strong worldwide, and this strength is largely a function of the longevity and enforceability of ethical standards in medicine. In various countries a proven commitment to medical ethics is a legal requirement to work as a clinician, and conduct deemed unethical can attract the professional sanction of the forfeit of permission to practice medicine. By contrast, there is currently no prospect of any individual scientist losing a "license" to conduct pathogen research. In the United States an ethos of professionalism among practitioners in this field is to an extent championed by organizations such as the American Society for Microbiology (ASM). A person's membership of the ASM can be terminated as a result of "conduct that is inimical to the objectives of the Society," although that person's livelihood is not thereby imperiled in the same way a medical doctor's is after being "struck off."[59] The ASM nevertheless aims to require and promote ethical behavior among its members, and one of the provisions in the society's 2005 code of ethics is "ASM members are obligated to discourage any use of microbiology contrary to the welfare of humankind, including the use of microbes as biological weapons."[60]

General exhortations of this kind stand in contrast, however, to the more detailed ethical guidance that is offered to medical practitioners by professional organizations like the American Medical Association. Moreover, short and broad statements of principle are likely to be of little assistance to a scientist who anticipates or encounters a dual-use dilemma while conducting pathogen research. Reasonable minds might differ, for example, on whether a particular activity is a "misuse" of microbiology or is "contrary to the welfare of humankind," and the ASM does not provide any guidance on how such determinations should be reached. The World Medical Association was similarly vague in its 2002 statement encouraging "all who participate in biomedical research to *consider* the implications and possible applications of their work and to *weigh carefully* in the balance the pursuit of scientific knowledge with their ethical responsibilities to society" (emphasis added).[61] If indeed such meager advice is an insufficient basis for reconciling the imperatives of scientific progress, national security, or public health, there is cause for pathogen researchers to collectively upgrade the role of ethics in their work and do so as a matter of professional interest and social responsibility. Specifically, as a way of navigating the secure or stifle dilemma, they could champion a code of ethics and integrate it into ongoing professional education. The idea of developing and promulgating such codes as a biosecurity governance measure is not new, but for the present discussion it is one worth reiterating. Despite widespread international support for such a code, progress to date has been slow, and the danger for pathogen researchers now is that wary governments might lose patience and impose yet more regulation.[62] As the WMD Commission warned in 2008:

The choice is stark. The life sciences community can wait until a catastrophic biological attack occurs before it steps up to its security responsibilities. Or it can act proactively in its own enlightened self-interest, aware that the reaction of the political system to a major bioterrorist event would likely be extreme and even draconian, resulting in significant harm to the scientific enterprise.[63]

Beyond "enlightened self-interest," being proactive on the matter of the dual-use dilemma would also enable pathogen researchers to shape the governance process into something beyond risk minimization. If codes of ethics promoted a process of carefully gauging the balance of risks *and* the benefits to be derived from research, scientists would be empowered to fulfill what is arguably a positive ethical obligation to society: to pursue and share lifesaving scientific discoveries.

There has been much debate about exactly what a code of ethics is and what its purpose should be, but it is commonly understood that a code is and should be distinct from a law.[64] That is, codes of ethics are intended generally to guide behavior (as a matter of professional responsibility) rather than mandate specific action (as a matter of legal obligation). One of the best examples of a code of ethics for pathogen researchers is the 2008 Code of Conduct on Biosecurity that was commissioned by the Royal Netherlands Academy of Arts and Sciences at the request of the Dutch Ministry of Education, Science, and Culture. Going beyond a general requirement not to misuse biotechnology, the Dutch code is more detailed in the guidance it offers, but as a short document (less than two pages long) it is also easy to understand and explain. The code begins with a statement of principle discouraging any use of microbiology contrary to the welfare of humankind, but it goes on to specify the kinds of people and organizations for whom the code is intended. Specific "rules of conduct" are then presented in categories, including raising awareness, research and publication policy, accountability and oversight, internal and external communication, accessibility, and shipment and transport. The research and publication policy rules, for example, are

- Screen for possible dual-use aspects during the application and assessment procedure and during the execution of research projects.
- Weigh the anticipated results against the risks of the research if possible dual-use aspects are identified.
- Reduce the risk that the publication of the results of potential dual-use life sciences research in scientific publications will unintentionally contribute to misuse of that knowledge.[65]

For all of its imprecision (what exactly does it mean, for example, to "screen" research?), the advantage of having a succinct code like this is that it could more readily induce pathogen researchers to consider—routinely and systematically—the balance of risks and benefits associated with a particular project. This would be a great step forward from a biosecurity governance perspective. Commitment to a code of ethics could be something shared among pathogen researchers worldwide, and a deepening of their professionalization could achieve governance traction on dual-use dilemmas where law-based regulation of laboratory research cannot.

CONCLUSION

The governance of laboratory-based pathogen research potentially gives rise to a biosecurity dilemma: secure or stifle. Measures designed by a government to make research practices more secure might make it less likely that pathogenic microorganisms will be used maliciously to harm. However, to the extent that such measures can stifle the pursuit of lifesaving scientific discoveries, the capacity for research-led protection against dreaded disease risks is undermined. Since the 2001 anthrax attacks, government efforts in the United States to reduce the risk of biological attacks from within have focused on allowing only "reliable" laboratory personnel access to particular microorganisms. By making it more difficult for a scientist-bioterrorist to act, some benefit is achieved in terms of health protection, but the regulation of pathogen research might also lead to lost opportunities. Despite the professional attractions of a boom in government-funded research for biodefense purposes, it is apparent that US biosecurity regulations are adversely affecting the ability and willingness of some scientists within and beyond the United States to discover new and better responses to infectious disease risks. On balance, US scientific capacity in this area could still increase over time. In any event, the counterproductive effect of increased laboratory regulations is but one dimension of the policy challenge that lies ahead. Even if these regulations are a necessary way of reducing the risk of biotechnology being misused, they are not sufficient alone and they fail to facilitate adequate consideration of the benefits that pathogen research can bring.

Beyond the reach of top-down, law-based approaches to the governance of laboratory biosecurity—such as the creation of lists of microorganisms or security clearances for scientists—pathogen researchers worldwide are likely to continue encountering dual-use dilemmas in their work. As a matter of professional ethics and in the public interest, pathogen researchers in general need to do a better job of considering the risks and benefits of their work in a timely and systematic fashion. One bottom-up approach to research governance that seems promising in this regard is the encouragement of individual and collective commitments to codes of ethics. Such codes could, from the moment a research project is conceived, be a constant point of reference for researchers. Although a code would not carry the force of law, it could serve as a governance measure that more readily affects the everyday practices of scientists. A code that is integral to professional identity could support an ongoing awareness of the problem of biological weapons from the time a would-be pathogen researcher began his or her education. It also could empower scientists to defend the potential of pathogen research to yield lifesaving discoveries against overzealous government regulators. This potential derives originally from the conduct of laboratory-based experiments, but the practical value of those experiments to public health is often critically dependent on the sharing of research findings. But here, too, a secure or stifle dilemma can arise. If the dissemination of biotechnology (both materials and techniques) can facilitate biological attacks perpetrated by its recipients, how should this practice be governed?

NOTES

1. Graham Allison et al., *World at Risk: The Report of the Commission on the Prevention of WMD Proliferation and Terrorism* (New York: Vintage, 2008), 11.
2. World Health Organization, "Laboratory Biosecurity Guidance," Report No. WHO/CDS/EPR/2006.6H, September 2006, http://www.who.int/csr/resources/publications/biosafety/WHO_CDS_EPR_2006_6.pdf?ua=1, 4.
3. "United States Code, Title 18, Part I, Chapter 10, Sec. 175 - Prohibitions with respect to biological weapons," US Government Printing Office, 2011, http://www.gpo.gov/fdsys/pkg/USCODE-2011-title18/html/USCODE-2011-title18-partI-chap10-sec175.htm.
4. Jennifer Gaudioso and Reynolds M. Salerno, "Biosecurity and Research: Minimizing Adverse Impacts," *Science* 304 (April 30, 2004): 687.
5. Federal Select Agent Program, "Select Agents and Toxins List," 2014, http://www.selectagents.gov/SelectAgentsandToxinsList.html.
6. "Uniting and Strengthening America by Providing Appropriate Tools Required to Intercept and Obstruct Terrorism (USA PATRIOT) Act of 2001," US Government Printing Office, 2001, http://www.gpo.gov/fdsys/pkg/PLAW-107publ56/html/PLAW-107publ56.htm, sec. 817.
7. "United States Code, Title 18, Part I, Chapter 10, Sec. 175b—Possession by restricted persons," US Government Printing Office, 2011. http://www.gpo.gov/fdsys/pkg/USCODE-2011-title18/html/USCODE-2011-title18-partI-chap10-sec175b.htm.
8. National Institutes of Health, "Enhancing Personnel Reliability among Individuals with Access to Select Agents," May 1, 2009, http://osp.od.nih.gov/sites/default/files/resources/NSABB%20Final%20Report%20on%20PR%205-29-09.pdf; National Research Council, *Responsible Research with Biological Select Agents and Toxins* (Washington, DC: National Academies Press, 2009); Kavita Marfatia Berger, Kathryn A. Luke, Mark S. Frankel, and Jennifer L. Sta. Ana, *Biological Safety Training Programs as a Component of Personnel Reliability: Workshop Report* (Washington, DC: American

Association for the Advancement of Science, 2009); National Research Council, *Beyond "Fortress America": National Security Controls on Science and Technology in a Globalized World* (Washington, DC: National Academies Press, 2009).

9. Federal Select Agent Program, "History," 2014, http://www.selectagents.gov/history.html.

10. Federal Select Agent Program, "Select Agents."

11. Yudhijit Bhattacharjee, "The Danger Within," *Science* 323 (March 6, 2009): 1282.

12. Ibid., 1283.

13. United States of America, "Key Biosecurity-Related Changes Made to the USA Select Agent Regulations," Report No. BWC/MSP/2013/MX/WP.4, United Nations Office at Geneva, July 29, 2013, http://repository.un.org/handle/11176/304348, 3.

14. Editorial, "The Case against Bruce Ivins," *Washington Post*, August 7, 2008, A20.

15. Yudhijit Bhattacharjee, "Army Missed Warning Signs about Alleged Anthrax Mailer," *Science* 332 (April 1, 2011): 27.

16. Nelson Hernandez and Philip Rucker, "Anthrax Case Raises Doubt in Security," *Washington Post*, August 8, 2008, A01.

17. National Institutes of Health, "Enhancing Personnel Reliability," iv.

18. National Research Council, *Globalization, Biosecurity, and the Future of the Life Sciences* (Washington, DC: National Academies Press, 2006), 8.

19. David R. Franz et al., "The 'Nuclearization' of Biology Is a Threat to Health and Security," *Biosecurity and Bioterrorism* 7, no. 3 (2009): 244.

20. M. Beatrice Dias, Leonardo Reyes-Gonzalez, Francisco M. Veloso, and Elizabeth A. Casman, "Effects of the USA PATRIOT Act and the 2002 Bioterrorism Preparedness Act on Select Agent Research in the United States," *Proceedings of the National Academy of Sciences* 107, no. 21 (2010): 9556.

21. Ibid., 9557; Heidi Ledford, "Regulations Increase Cost of Dangerous-Pathogen Research," *Nature*, May 10, 2010, http://www.nature.com/news/2010/100510/full/news.2010.231.html.

22. Erika Check, "Law Sends Laboratories into Pathogen Panic," *Nature* 421 (January 2, 2003): 4.

23. Frank Gottron and Dana A. Shea, *Oversight of High-Containment Biological Laboratories: Issues for Congress* (Washington, DC: Congressional Research Service, 2009), 3.

24. Arturo Casadevall and Michael J. Imperiale, "Destruction of Microbial Collections in Response to Select Agent and Toxin List Regulations," *Biosecurity and Bioterrorism* 8, no. 2 (2010): 152.

25. Ibid.

26. Judith Miller, "New Germ Labs Stir Debate Over Secrecy and Safety," *New York Times*, February 10, 2004, F1.

27. Charles Piller, "Plague Expert Cleared of Serious Charges in Bioterror Case," *Los Angeles Times*, December 2, 2003, A16.

28. Kenneth Chang, "Scientist in Plague Case Is Sentenced to Two Years," *New York Times*, March 11, 2004, 18; Piller, "Plague Expert Cleared," A16.

29. For an extended discussion of this case, see Christian Enemark, *Disease and Security: Natural Plagues and Biological Weapons in East Asia* (Abingdon, UK: Routledge, 2007), 146–49.

30. See Victoria Sutton, "Survey Finds Biodefense Researcher Anxiety over Inadvertently Violating Regulations," *Biosecurity and Bioterrorism* 7, no. 2 (2009): 225–26.

31. Julie E. Fischer, *Stewardship or Censorship? Balancing Biosecurity, the Public's Health, and the Benefits of Scientific Openness* (Washington, DC: Henry L. Stimson Center, 2006), 64.

32. Declan Butler, "Viral Research Faces Clampdown," *Nature* 490 (October 25, 2012): 456.

33. Kavita M. Berger et al., *Bridging Science and Security for Biological Research International Science and Security* (Washington, DC: American Association for the Advancement of Science, 2013).

34. Laurie Garrett, "Biology's Brave New World: The Promise and Perils of the Synbio Revolution," *Foreign Affairs* (November–December 2013): 40.

35. National Research Council, *Globalization, Biosecurity*, 4–5.

36. National Research Council, *Science and Security in a Post-9/11 World: A Report Based on Regional Discussions between the Science and Security Communities* (Washington, DC: National Academies Press, 2007), 3.

37. National Research Council, *Beyond "Fortress America,"* 10.

38. See, for example, David P. Fidler and Lawrence O. Gostin, *Biosecurity in the Global Age: Biological Weapons, Public Health, and the Rule of Law* (Stanford, CA: Stanford University Press, 2008), 85.

39. See, for example, Roger Roffey and Chandré Gould, "Preventing Misuse of the Life Sciences: The Need to Improve Biodefense Transparency and Accountability in the BWC," *Nonproliferation Review* 18, no. 3 (2011): 558.

40. Bob Graham and Jim Talent, "Bioterrorism: Redefining Prevention," *Biosecurity and Bioterrorism* 7, no. 2 (2009): 126.

41. National Research Council, *Biotechnology Research in an Age of Terrorism* (Washington, DC: National Academy of Sciences, 2004), 5.

42. US Department of Health and Human Services, "United States Government Policy for Oversight of Life Sciences Dual Use Research of Concern," March 2012, http://www.phe.gov/s3/dualuse/Documents/us-policy-durc-032812.pdf.

43. Terrence M. Tumpey et al., "Characterization of the Reconstructed 1918 Spanish Influenza Pandemic Virus," *Science* 310, no. 5745 (2005): 77–80.

44. See Andreas von Bubnoff, "The 1918 Flu Virus Is Resurrected," *Nature* 437 (October 6, 2005): 794–95.

45. Masaki Imai et al., "Experimental Adaptation of an Influenza H5 HA Confers Respiratory Droplet Transmission to a Reassortant H5 HA/H1N1 Virus in Ferrets," *Nature* 486 (June 21, 2012): 420–28.

46. Sander Herfst et al., "Airborne Transmission of Influenza A/H5N1 Virus between Ferrets," *Science* 336 (June 22, 2012): 1534–41.

47. Brendan Maher, "The Biosecurity Oversight," *Nature* 485 (May 24, 2012): 432.

48. Yoshihiro Kawaoka, "Flu Transmission Work Is Urgent," *Nature* (February 9, 2012): 155.

49. Marc Lipsitch and Alison P. Galvani, "Ethical Alternatives to Experiments with Novel Potential Pandemic Pathogens," *PLoS Medicine* (May 20, 2014), http://journals.plos.org/plosmedicine/article?id=10.1371/journal.pmed.1001646.

50. Ibid.

51. Ian Sample, "Virus Experiments Risk Unleashing Global Pandemic, Study Warns," *Guardian* (London), May 21, 2014, http://www.theguardian.com/world/2014/may/20/virus-experiments-risk-global-pandemic.

52. Veronika Hackenbroch and Gerald Traufetter, "Containing Super-Flus: Controversy Brews over Scientists' Creation of Killer Viruses," *Der Spiegel*, February 17, 2012, http://www.spiegel.de/international/spiegel/containing-super-flus-controversy-brews-over-scientists-creation-of-killer-viruses-a-815782-2.html.

53. David Murphy, "Lab Bungle," *Far Eastern Economic Review* (May 6, 2004): 18; Jim Yardley and Lawrence K. Altman, "China Is Scrambling to Curb SARS Cases after a Death," *New York Times*, April 24, 2004, 4.

54. Ron A.M. Fouchier et al., "Pause on Avian Flu Transmission Studies," *Nature* 481 (January 26, 2012): 443.

55. White House Office of Science and Technology Policy, "Doing Diligence to Assess the Risks and Benefits of Life Sciences Gain-of-Function Research," October 17, 2014, http://www.whitehouse.gov/blog/2014/10/17/doing-diligence-assess-risks-and-benefits-life-sciences-gain-function-research.

56. Sara Reardon, "Viral-Research Moratorium Called Too Broad," *Nature* (October 23, 2014), http://www.nature.com/news/viral-research-moratorium-called-too-broad-1.16211.

57. United Nations Office at Geneva, "Report of the Meeting of States Parties," Report No. BWC/MSP/2008/5, December 12, 2008, http://repository.un.org/handle/11176/280410, 7.

58. Samuel P. Huntington, *The Soldier and the State: The Theory and Politics of Civil-Military Relations* (Cambridge, MA: Harvard University Press, 1957), 10.

59. American Society for Microbiology, "Constitution and Bylaws," n.d., http://www.asm.org/index.php/governance/constitution-and-bylaws.

60. American Society for Microbiology, "Code of Ethics," 2005, http://www.asm.org/ccLibraryFiles/FILENAME/000000001596/ASMCodeofEthics05.pdf.

61. World Medical Association, "WMA Declaration of Washington on Biological Weapons," October 2002, http://www.wma.net/en/30publications/10policies/b1/.

62. See United Nations Office at Geneva, "Final Document of the Seventh Review Conference" Report No. BWC/CONF.VII/7 (January 13, 2012), http://www.unog.ch/80256EDD006B8954/%28httpAssets%29/3E2A1AA4CF86184BC1257D960032AA4E/$file/BWC_CONF.VII_07+%28E%29.pdf, 11

63. Allison et al., *World at Risk*, 26.

64. See Brian Rappert, "Codes of Conduct and Biological Weapons: An In-Process Assessment," *Biosecurity and Bioterrorism* 5, no. 2 (2007): 145–54.

65. Royal Netherlands Academy of Arts and Sciences, "A Code of Conduct on Biosecurity: Report by the Biosecurity Working Group," August 2008, https://www.knaw.nl/en/news/publications/a-code-of-conduct-for-biosecurity.

4

EXPORT AND PUBLICATION CONTROLS

THE PRACTICE OF LIMITING scientists' physical access to the pathogenic microorganisms that cause dreaded diseases could reduce the risk of biological attacks. It could also reduce the likelihood of scientific discoveries that assist the protection of population health in the event of an outbreak of natural or deliberate origin. However, the scope of this secure or stifle dilemma extends beyond the scientific work that goes on inside a laboratory. After the moment of scientific discovery, biosecurity governance can involve efforts to restrict access by controlling the transfer of pathogen samples between scientists. It also can involve controls on the sharing of information that shows how a pathogen with particular genetic characteristics could be produced. Increasingly, the granting of access to pathogens is less about the transport of physical material (organisms and related equipment) and more about the transfer of intangible technology (techniques and methods applied at the molecular level). The latter occurs on a larger scale when the description of a technique used in an experiment is published in a widely read, peer-reviewed scientific journal. This chapter focuses on the use of experimental technologies of genetic engineering and synthetic genomics and is concerned primarily with publication as an intangible form of technology-transfer. The analysis is presented in two sections: the first explores the tension between the governance imperatives of restrictiveness and permissiveness when it comes to the sharing of dual-use biotechnology, with particular concern for export-control regulations and publication decisions by journal editors; the second discusses the legal and ethical questions surrounding the 2012 publication in *Science* of findings from controversial research on influenza virus transmissibility. This research involved genetic manipulation of the H5N1 bird flu virus into a potentially pandemic form. The chapter then concludes by recommending a policy of "discreet dissemination" of pathogen research findings as an alternative to censorship in cases where a secure or stifle dilemma arises. Such a policy would involve the withholding of particular findings from general distribution (e.g., via a scientific journal) while nevertheless making those findings available to scientists who, for public health purposes, need them.

DUAL-USE BIOTECHNOLOGY AND EXPORT CONTROLS

During the study of microorganisms by molecular biologists around the world, the technology transferred among researchers is often and increasingly not tangible but intangible. Experiments on microorganisms undertaken at the molecular level that result in genetically mutated microbes are carried out in laboratory settings, and generally the standard scientific practice is to share a description of how the mutation was achieved with other scientists. Sharing takes the form of presentations at conferences, emails to colleagues, lectures to students, postings on websites, or the publication of research findings in a journal. Sometimes the technology thereby transferred is a method for creating a "new" microorganism (i.e., one different from its forms known in nature) that is more dangerous to humans (more transmissible, more virulent, more resistant to a vaccine, etc.). This sharing process, in addition to being a professional expectation for both peer review and quality-control purposes, has the potential to improve public health efforts and thus benefit populations worldwide. By being better informed about the potential dangerousness of a pathogen that could mutate naturally "in the wild," other scientists and governments could develop pharmaceutical and other means for defending against it. At the same time there is a concern that publishing information on *how* to make a pathogen more dangerous (in a laboratory setting) could encourage and enable the application of that knowledge for offensive (biological weapon) purposes.

Biological attacks are universally prohibited, and Article I of the BWC binds member states never to develop, produce, stockpile, or otherwise acquire or retain "microbial or other biological agents, or toxins whatever their origin or method of production, of types and in quantities that have no justification for prophylactic, protective or other peaceful purposes." Article IV requires states to affirm this rule within their domestic laws. However, the great difficulty is to discern reliably the *lack* of a "justification for . . . peaceful purposes," given the importance of biomedical research to human health and the scale of the scientific enterprise directed toward understanding microorganisms. The task of preventing the use of microorganisms in attacks is also made difficult, legally speaking, by two BWC provisions between which there is clear tension. On the one hand Article III of the convention requires member states "not to transfer to any recipient whatsoever, directly or indirectly, and not in any way to assist, encourage, or induce" the manufacture or acquisition of any "[biological] agents" specified in Article I.

On the other hand, Article X requires states to "facilitate . . . the fullest possible exchange" of technology and to "cooperate in contributing . . . to the further development and application of scientific discoveries in the field of bacteriology (biology) for prevention of disease, or for other peaceful purposes."[1]

The language of Article X ("peaceful purposes") is such that the provision is subject to interpretations of intent, and it has long been a sign of international distrust that developed countries are afraid to share certain kinds of biotechnology with developing countries for fear that it will not be used for peaceful purposes only. At the 2011 BWC Review Conference the language used in the final consensus statement did little to reduce the tension between the nonproliferation and the technology-transfer imperatives of the convention:

> the Conference urges all States Parties possessing advanced biotechnology to adopt positive measures to promote technology transfer and international cooperation on an equal and non-discriminatory basis, particularly with countries less advanced in this field, while promoting the basic objectives of the Convention, as well as *ensuring that the promulgation of science and technology is fully consistent with the peaceful object and purpose of the Convention.* (emphasis added)[2]

The political effort to ensure "full consistency" has traditionally included the imposition of export controls, which reflects the tendency of many developed countries to favor an emphasis on reducing proliferation risks over facilitating technology transfers. The potential ethical problem with this, though, is that any technological deprivation caused by export controls might have a greater adverse impact on public health in a developing country than on that country's capacity to maintain a biological weapons program. Since 1984 a group of states known as the Australia Group (AG) has cooperated to restrict exports of biological (and chemical) technologies with a view to preventing their use in weaponized form. However, among many developing countries these restrictions are perceived as "unfair trade barriers and an attempt by an exclusive club of rich countries to prevent technological developments elsewhere in the world."[3] The AG maintains a series of lists that define dual-use biological agents and biological equipment; participating states are informally committed to ensuring these items are subjected to national export controls, and each state assesses export license applications in accordance with an agreed-on set of guidelines.[4] The list of controlled equipment includes, for example, fermenters, aerosol inhalation chambers, and spraying systems. In the category of "related technology," controls are intended to cover the "transfer of technology (technical data) by any means, including electronic media, fax or telephone" as well as the "transfer of technology in the form of technical assistance," though there is an exception for "basic scientific research."[5]

The decision to control "the intangible transfer of information and knowledge" was made at an AG meeting in 2002, but the implementation of enforceable legislation by participating states has occurred relatively recently.[6] For example, in 2012 the Australian government implemented the Defence Trade Controls Act, according to which any person who commits an offense may be imprisoned for ten years if he or she "supplies DSGL [Defence and Strategic Goods List] technology to another person . . . outside Australia" without a permit issued by the minister for defence.[7] The minister may issue a permit when "satisfied that the supply [of DSGL technology] would not prejudice the security, defence or international relations of Australia."[8] The DSGL (which includes more than one hundred pathogens) refers to "genetically modified organisms or genetic elements that contain nucleic acid sequences associated with pathogenicity of organisms."[9] Regarding intangible technology transfers, a regulatory impact statement by the Australian government assessed that the legislation "should have minimal impact on . . . research programs as these controls will not apply to broad *discussions* of research projects or experiments that do not *discuss* or transfer technology listed in the DSGL" (emphasis added).[10] Nevertheless, the legislation induced fear among some Australian scientists who worried that the new requirement for an export permit would inhibit their ability to communicate with international colleagues electronically, in-person at conferences, or via the publication of research findings.[11]

The regulatory reach of another AG participant, the European Union (EU), is similar to that of Australia. Since 2009, the EU's Council Regulation 428/2009 has provided a regime for controlling exports of dual-use technology by EU member states to non-EU states. When an item of dual-use technology (such as a microorganism) is listed in Annex 1 of the regulation, the member state must require the export of that item to be officially authorized. The regulation defines "export" to include

> transmission of software or technology by electronic media, including by fax, telephone, electronic mail or any other electronic means to a destination outside the European Community; it includes making available in an electronic form such software and technology to legal and natural persons and partnerships outside the Community. Export also applies to oral transmission of technology when the technology is described over the telephone.[12]

For example, authorization is required for emailing (to a recipient outside the EU) information describing an experiment that uses a listed microorganism unless the experiment is "basic scientific research."[13] Electronic submission of a manuscript to an international journal with a view to electronic publication worldwide thus appears to be covered by the regulation. (A later section of this chapter will discuss a legal dispute that arose in the Netherlands over the applicability of the "basic research" exception.) It is important to consider more generally why a government might wish, for biosecurity reasons, to control the dissemination of scientific findings in the field of pathogen research.

Increasingly, and as a result of scientific advances in genetic engineering and gene synthesis, microorganisms expressing certain genes can be produced in a laboratory. Consequently, scientists with the necessary skill can achieve possession of a microorganism with certain characteristics by acquiring and applying the method of its production. A step-by-step description of that method could be conveyed directly from one scientist to another, or it could be shared indirectly and on a wide scale. Dissemination of research findings (including the experimental techniques used in the research) occurs on an intermediate scale via conferences attended by many scientists and via project websites accessible to many more. But the most extensive form of dissemination is publication in a respected journal that is read widely. In terms of research impact, journal publication affords scientific discoveries the greatest exposure and so increases the chance that findings will be used for positive benefits (e.g., in the case of pathogen research, to improve human health). At the same time, the wide-scale dissemination of a scientific method also increases the likelihood that an ill-intentioned or reckless scientist will acquire and apply it in a way that causes harm. In a small number of cases the risk of harmful application of published methods has been perceived by some as unacceptably high, relative to the benefit of publication. The controversy surrounding these cases has in turn gradually intensified the political pressure on journal editors to refrain from publishing or else see governments take the decision out of their hands.

One such controversy arose from an article that appeared in the *Journal of Virology* in 2001, just prior to the anthrax attacks in the United States. In the article, a group of scientists from Australia described research showing that mousepox virus expressing the spliced-in *interleukin-4* gene was much more deadly than unmodified mousepox and was able to kill even vaccinated mice.[14] A disturbing implication was that applying this gene-addition method might similarly increase the virulence of *variola major* (smallpox) and potentially allow that virus too to circumvent vaccination. Questioned by the *New York Times* on the decision to publish and the biological weapons risk that publishing posed, project leader Ron Jackson said, "We thought it was better that the information came out in case somebody constructed something more sinister. . . . We felt we had a moral obligation because it is existing technology."[15] A fellow Australian scientist, Bob

Seamark, applauded such awareness-raising: "The best protection against any mis-use of this technique was to issue a worldwide warning."[16] But D. A. Henderson, who led the global campaign to eradicate smallpox from nature, took a dimmer view. Referring to the problem that "blueprints for making microorganisms more harmful" were appearing in unclassified journals, he told *New Scientist* magazine: "I can't for the life of me figure out how we are going to deal with this."[17]

The following year, in the aftermath of the US anthrax attacks, another "blue-print" article appeared. It was authored by some US scientists sponsored by the US Defense Department who had spent three years chemically synthesizing the *poliomyelitis* (polio) virus. Referring to the published virus genome, they had strung together corresponding sequences of genetic material purchased via the Internet. The assembled material was then used to create live polio virus that paralyzed and killed mice. The 2002 publication of this finding in *Science* showed that eradicating a virus in the wild might not mean it is gone forever.[18] More broadly, the findings demonstrated how synthesis technology can obviate the need to source pathogens from natural reservoirs or from other laboratories. The leader of the research team, Eckard Wimmer, later told the *Washington Post*: "To most scientists and lay people, the reality that viruses could be synthesized was surprising, if not shocking. We consider it imperative to inform society of this new reality, which bears far-reaching consequences."[19] Criticism of the decision to publish ranged from arguments that the research findings were scientifically uninteresting to arguments that the information could be maliciously and harm-fully misused by readers. One US congressman even tabled a congressional reso-lution accusing *Science* of publishing "a blueprint that could conceivably enable terrorists to inexpensively create human pathogens."[20] But the journal's editor, Donald Kennedy, defended the decision by arguing, "Sticking one's head in the sand and hoping that unpleasant realities will go away has never been a fruit-ful approach to science or public policy." He conceded, nevertheless, that "there should continue to be serious conversations about the relationship between sci-entific research, publication, and security."[21]

Six months later Kennedy was one of the thirty-two journal editors and authors who published a "Statement on the Consideration of Biodefence and Biosecurity" in *Nature*. The statement in February 2003 was in part a response to "questions . . . asked . . . by some political leaders about the possibility that new information published in research journals might give aid to those with malevolent ends." It acknowledged that "there is information that, although we cannot now capture it with lists of definitions, presents enough risk of use by ter-rorists that it should not be published." At the same time, the statement's authors considered it vital to "protect the integrity of the scientific process by publishing manuscripts of high quality, in sufficient detail to permit reproducibility." The rationale for this was couched in both scientific and security terms: without the independent verification required for scientific progress, "we can neither advance biomedical research nor provide the knowledge base for building strong biodefence systems." Accordingly, this group of editors and authors announced that they would henceforth weigh the potential harm of publication against the scientific benefits of a submitted research article and make the decision to modify or publish manuscripts on that basis.[22] On its own the assurance did not appear to be sufficient from the perspective of the US government. The following year the Department of Health and Human Services (DHHS) established the National Science Advisory Board for Biosecurity (NSABB) composed of twenty-five non-government experts, one role of which was to "advise on strategies to work with journal editors and other stakeholders to ensure the development of guidelines for the publication, public presentation, and public communication of potentially sensitive life sciences research."[23]

In 2005 journal editors again came under political pressure over three published papers, each of which carried the potential both to address and to generate biosecurity risks. The first paper did not describe pathogen research undertaken at the molecular level, but it is significant for present purposes because its authors relied on an "awareness-raising" justification similar to Jackson's (viz. mousepox) and Wimmer's (viz. polio). The paper modeled an attack involving the deliberate contamination of the US milk supply with botulinum toxin (derived from *Clostridium botulinum* bacteria), and both estimated the extent of illness and death that would result and spelled out what steps the government and industry could take to prevent such an attack.[24] Soon after the DHHS learned of the paper's imminent publication in *Proceedings of the National Academy of Sciences*, officials made an unprecedented request to the journal not to publish. As the paper was "a road map for terrorists," publication would be perceived as "not in the interests of the United States."[25] The journal nevertheless proceeded with publication.[26] In a covering editorial, National Academy of Sciences president Bruce Alberts explained that publication was justified because "all of the critical information in this article that could be useful to a terrorist . . . are immediately accessible on the World Wide Web through a simple Google search."[27]

A pair of papers describing research on the 1918 Spanish flu virus was published in late 2005 (one in *Nature* and the other in *Science*), but the government—which had funded the research—first referred the manuscripts to the NSABB for advice on whether the benefit of the future use of this information outweighed the potential risk of misuse.[28] In combination, the findings revealed (and reproduced in animals) the genetic traits that made this influenza virus so deadly and able to kill around 50 million people worldwide in 1918–19. The promise of sharing such information was that it could assist in further gene-synthesis experiments aimed at better understanding the nature of influenza viruses and the development of new vaccines or treatments. However, the publication of this information also gave rise to concerns that would-be bioterrorists could use it to reconstruct the virus for the purpose of attacking a target population with no natural immunity. An article in the *New York Times*, for example, described the published genome of the 1918 influenza virus as "essentially the design of a weapon of mass destruction."[29] Nevertheless, members of the NSABB quickly agreed that publication should proceed anyway, while *Science*'s Donald Kennedy responded that the risk of doing so was far outweighed by the benefit that it "could help prevent another global flu pandemic."[30] The editor of *Nature*, Philip Campbell, agreed with Kennedy, although in reflecting on the NSABB's involvement, he warned, "Government bureaucracies and committees may push to avoid perceived risks, at the potential expense of benefits to public security."[31]

Reminiscent of Campbell's warning, another crisis erupted six years later, and again the object of concern was a pair of papers describing influenza virus research. Although the publication of one paper each in *Science* and *Nature* ultimately went ahead, the paper submitted to *Science* is worthy of special consideration because it came closest to being government censored on biosecurity grounds. Accordingly, the next section explores the ethical question of whether publication of that paper was justified.

HOW TO MAKE A VIRUS MUTATE: THE ETHICS OF PUBLICATION

A severe pandemic of influenza is a public health risk of global concern. As against that risk, protection of human health is in large measure dependent on a strong scientific understanding of the properties and behavior of influenza viruses. For this reason, laboratory-based influenza research, to the extent that it potentially contributes to better treatments and disease-control methods, is important to all people everywhere. Moreover, the more quickly scientific discoveries can be accumulated and communicated prior to the next influenza pandemic, the more potential there might be for those discoveries to contribute to the saving of lives. When time is of the essence, research results that are predictive of future influenza risk appear to be particularly valuable, assuming adequate capacity exists to erect public health defenses. Preempting the natural genetic mutation of influenza viruses into a form more dangerous to humans is one such avenue of inquiry. Accordingly, scientists worldwide have speculated for some time that, by "reassorting" (mixing) avian influenza viruses with human influenza viruses in the laboratory, they could discover how dangerous the hybrid virus would be and gauge the likelihood of it igniting a pandemic.

In 2011 a breakthrough occurred when one team of scientists in the Netherlands and another in the United States managed to cause the mutation of H5N1 avian influenza virus into a form directly transmissible (through the air) between ferrets. A ferret's respiratory system closely resembles that of a human, and ferret-to-ferret transmission of influenza virus is generally understood to demonstrate human-to-human transmissibility. This meant that a new and presumably human-to-human transmissible influenza virus subtype had emerged not through natural processes but as a result of human experimentation. A manuscript describing Yoshihiro Kawaoka's US-based team's process for achieving the virus's "gain of function" was prepared for publication in *Nature*, while Ron Fouchier's team in the Netherlands prepared a similar manuscript for *Science*. In December 2011 the NSABB (to which the journals' editors had referred the manuscripts) recommended against publishing both sets of findings unless certain methodological details were omitted. The recommendation was unanimous, and one board member told the *New York Times* "My concern is that we don't give amateurs—or terrorists—information that might let them do something that could really cause a lot of harm."[32] Three months later, after considering revised papers from each research team, the NSABB recommended that both should be published, although one-third of the board's voting members remained opposed to the publication of Fouchier's findings.[33] Meanwhile, because *Science* is based (and can be read) outside the EU, the Dutch government decided, pursuant to EU Regulation 428/2009, that Fouchier first needed to apply for and receive an export permit.[34] For the first time, as a matter of biosecurity practice as well as law, a government had conceptualized publication as exportation. A permit was in fact applied for and granted (in April 2012), and publication went ahead, although Fouchier subsequently went to court twice to question the legality of requiring such a permit in the first place.[35]

The Legal Issue: "Basic" vs. "Applied" Research

Article 3.1 of Regulation 428/2009 provides that "authorisation shall be required for the export of the dual-use items listed in Annex I," and the annex lists highly pathogenic avian influenza viruses of subtype H5. Controls on "technology" transfer do not apply to "basic scientific research," and the regulation defines the latter as "experimental or theoretical work undertaken principally to acquire new knowledge of the fundamental principles of phenomena . . . not primarily directed towards a specific practical aim or objective."[36] Given that the primary purpose of the regulation is nonproliferation (of weapons), the Dutch government might simply have decided that it was more prudent to err on the side of caution and assume that the regulation's basic-research exemption did not apply. In later opposing the imposition of a requirement for an export permit in respect of his findings on H5N1 influenza, Fouchier's legal argument was that he had engaged in basic scientific research. The ferret studies were basic, he reasoned, because the researchers sought to better understand mammalian transmissibility of an influenza strain. An alternative view is that research is "basic" only if it is directed toward greater understanding of the fundamental aspects of phenomena without specific applications in mind. Yet, beyond the impetus of simple curiosity, there appears to have been a public-spirited motivation behind Fouchier's research. In the article that eventually appeared in *Science*, the authors explained, "To address *the concern* that the virus could acquire [airborne transmission] ability under natural conditions, we genetically modified A/H5N1 virus by . . ." (emphasis added).[37] A subsequent claim by Kawaoka about Fouchier's research made it appear even more to be of a non-"basic" kind and rather "directed towards a specific practical aim or objective," to use the language of Regulation 428/2009:

> the ferret transmission studies in my lab and Ron Fouchier's lab demonstrated that H5N1 viruses have pandemic potential and it is important to continue to stockpile H5N1 vaccines. This is a critical point since vaccines expire and decisions by policy makers as to whether we continue to stockpile H5N1 vaccines should be based on scientific facts.[38]

In September 2013 the District Court of Noord-Holland in Haarlem rejected Fouchier's argument and upheld the government's decision to characterize Fouchier's intended transfer of intangible technology (that is, publication of research findings) as an export covered by Regulation 428/2009. The court held that the government had correctly interpreted EU regulations aimed at preventing the proliferation of WMD and dual-use technology, and making H5N1 airborne was a practical goal rather than basic research. The court's justification was that the regulation's exceptions "should be interpreted strictly" and that it is not up to individual researchers to decide whether their work is basic research.[39] When Fouchier appealed the decision, however, the Dutch Court of Appeal in Amsterdam held (nearly two years later) that it did not need to decide whether his research was "basic" or "applied" and thus whether the transfer of resulting data was subject to EU export regulations. Rather, that court was able to dismiss the appeal on the issue of legal standing alone: Fouchier, after applying to the Dutch government for an export permit, no longer had a legal entitlement to dispute the requirement to do so.[40] In neither case did the court address the more interesting and difficult *ethical* question, Assuming the Dutch government was legally correct in requiring a permit application, was the granting of permission for Fouchier to send his article to *Science* the right thing to do?

The Ethical Issue: Weighing Benefits and Risks

It is not clear why the Dutch government granted a permit for Fouchier to transfer his intangible technology to the editor of *Science*, but its decision set a precedent for government control of the transfer of intangible technology. Future decisions will need to be made on a principled basis, and it would be unfair for a government decision maker to withhold authorization for a publication-as-export on the basis that transferring a particular technology *might in some way* pose a risk. Doing so would be to likewise discount the possibility of any benefit and thereby deny the characterization of items subject to export controls as truly *dual* use. A better approach would be to weigh carefully the likely risks *and* benefits of publishing research findings and to permit publication when the benefits are assessed as clearly outweighing the risks.

Such an approach could take its inspiration from, for example, the principles that constitute the 1947 Nuremberg Code. These principles are concerned primarily with the requirement for informed consent from human subjects of medical research, though the code does not explicitly account for the possible ramifications of research. However, one principle is that "the experiment should be such as to yield fruitful results *for the good of society*"; another is that "the degree of risk to be taken should never exceed that determined by the *humanitarian importance of the problem* to be solved by the experiment" (emphases added).[41] The first principle suggests the need to apply to research a "some benefit" values test; the second implies that the risk associated with research should generally be less than (and never more than) the benefit. The notion that risk and benefit must be weighed for the purposes of ethical judgment is further reflected in principles for preventing hostile use of the life sciences, as published by the International Committee on the Red Cross in 2004. Underpinning these is the "general principle" that "the benefits to humanity of any particular development in the life sciences must always outweigh the risks of that development being used to facilitate poisoning and deliberate spread of infectious disease."[42] Such a principle, concerned as it is with the *application* of technology, seems eminently suitable as a basis for assessing the ethics of publishing research findings and thereby sharing techniques with other scientists.

What, then, were the benefits and risks that the Dutch government might have considered in deciding whether to grant Ron Fouchier an export permit in 2012? The main argument in favor of publication was that it would, on balance, be good for public health. At a WHO workshop held in February 2012, the consensus among the technical experts participating was that "influenza A(H5N1) viruses remain an important risk for causing a future pandemic" and that "the results of [Fouchier's and Kawaoka's] studies provide an important contribution to public health surveillance of H5N1 viruses and to a better understanding of the properties of these viruses." The participants acknowledged the safety and security risks of conducting research on influenza virus transmissibility. Regarding the issue of disseminating research findings, however, they had "a preference, from a public health perspective, for full disclosure of the information in these papers."[43] The following month, when the NSABB considered a revised manuscript submitted by Fouchier, twelve of the eighteen voting members of the board recommended the full communication of the Dutch team's data, methods, and conclusions. The benefit of publication was couched in the following terms:

> New evidence has emerged that underscores the fact that understanding specific mutations may improve international surveillance and public health and safety. Global cooperation, critical for pandemic influenza preparedness efforts, is predicated upon the free sharing of information and was a fundamental principle in evaluating these manuscripts.[44]

Prior to this NSABB meeting, Fouchier himself had made his own argument in a televised interview:

> We have to be prepared for such viruses to emerge in the wild. If we would detect these viruses out in the field, then we could go out to outbreak areas and try to eradicate the virus and prevent a pandemic from happening. If that would fail, then we would still be in a good position to, ahead of that pandemic, evaluate our vaccines and anti-viral drugs and therefore gain months of time if a pandemic would hit and therefore we would be able to handle it better.[45]

However, the public health benefit of publishing research findings on influenza virus mutation is diminished, in practice, if systemic problems deny the theoretical opportunity to "prevent a pandemic from happening." On the issue of translating scientific discoveries into actual benefits, six of the eighteen NSABB members who attended the March 2012 meeting concluded that "the current [disease] surveillance infrastructure is ill-equipped to detect the emergence of highly transmissible influenza viruses in real time prior to their dissemination in nature."[46] NSABB chairman Paul Keim earlier observed "Even if we did spot [an emerging influenza virus] early on, I don't think we have sufficient vaccines.

The vaccines aren't good enough, and the drugs are not good enough to stop this emerging and being a pandemic."[47] The message here seemed to be that the benefit of publication—to inform scientists worldwide of a molecular-level discovery—is dependent on the degree to which the information can be exploited at the system level by public health practitioners. If the prospect of beneficial application of published findings is slim, it is harder to claim that any risk associated with publication is outweighed.

Just as it is possible to overestimate the practical benefit(s) to be derived from publishing dual-use pathogen research findings, so too is it possible to overestimate the risk that publication will result in harm. The view of a minority of NSABB members in March 2012 was that "the revised Fouchier manuscript provides information that would enable the near-term misuse of the research in ways that would endanger public health or national security."[48] However, the degree of endangerment would depend first on the extent to which a deliberately mutated, pandemic version of H5N1 influenza virus could cause illness and death. On the one hand it is cause for concern that, since 2003, H5N1 has had a global average case-fatality rate of around 53 percent.[49] On the other hand, it is worth noting that, in Fouchier's experiments, "none of the recipient ferrets died after airborne infection with the mutant A/H5N1 viruses."[50] This is consistent with the generally observed phenomenon that a virus's virulence decreases as its transmissibility increases. A second consideration for risk assessors is whether scientists other than those working in Fouchier's laboratory really could achieve possession of his mutated H5N1 virus simply by following the published procedure for creating it. That is, to what extent (if at all) has publication increased the accessibility of this organism? In 2002, when Eckard Wimmer's team published its polio virus synthesis technique, doing so did not increase accessibility to that organism to a high degree. As one of Wimmer's colleagues, Aniko Paul, later explained, "For terrorists, it would have made no sense to start putting this virus together because they already had an ample supply of poliovirus available. Polio is present in old medical samples that are stored in freezers, and it can still be bought from suppliers."[51] By contrast, a human-to-human transmissible H5N1 virus is not readily available, so information on how to create one is nearly the sole determinant of access.

When Kawaoka responded to the NSABB's initial recommendation against publishing his and Fouchier's findings, he argued that "there is already enough information publicly available to allow someone to make a transmissible H5 HA-possessing virus."[52] The implication was that publication generated no additional risk. However, the problem with the "already out there" argument is that the publication of a particular piece of writing is not simply an exercise in data dissemination; it also serves the purpose of assembling and synthesizing diffuse information *for* the reader. It can otherwise take considerable time and skill to bring together ideas and information from various sources and to craft them into an integrated, clearly explained message. Thus, on the matter of "allow[ing] someone to make a transmissible H5 HA-possessing virus," publication of Fouchier's (and Kawaoka's) findings might have served *qualitatively* to increase accessibility to the necessary mutation technology. Nevertheless, in respect of any "recipe," there remains the possibility that it will not be followed correctly or that a key "ingredient" will unknowingly be left out. On the issue of biological weapons proliferation, for example, Sonia Ben Ouagrham-Gormley has found that "such intangible factors as organizational makeup and management style greatly affect the use of acquired knowledge" and that these factors "cannot be easily transferred among individuals or from one place to another."[53] If this is true of "proliferation" in the realm of pathogen research more generally (in the form of publication of methodologies), it is perhaps cause to afford less weight to the risk of information being harmfully misused.

CONCLUSION: THE CASE FOR "DISCREET DISSEMINATION"

Had the Dutch government in 2012 engaged in a process of reasoning regarding Fouchier's H5N1 findings in a way similar to that described above, it could have reasonably concluded that the risks of publication outweighed the benefits and that authorization for an export permit should be withheld. The government's actual conclusion to the contrary could also have been a reasonable one, although in both instances the morally correct decision would probably not have been obvious. The prospect of an intangible transfer of technology thus presented a secure or stifle biosecurity dilemma for Dutch decision makers: protection against the dreaded risk of an influenza pandemic seemed to necessitate both a permissive approach *and* a restrictive one. The duality of the uses to which Fouchier's virus-mutation technology might be put (good and evil) appeared to induce a strictly binary approach to policy: publication or nonpublication. However, this need not be the case in the future. Arguably, when faced with the challenge of satisfying simultaneously the nonproliferation and technology-transfer imperatives of biosecurity policy, a middle way deserves to be tried: the "discreet dissemination" of research findings. It is an approach to biosecurity governance that would afford governments and scientists an alternative to the extremes of unfettered publication and outright censorship.

Government decision-making might sometimes be preempted by self-censoring scientists, although it is difficult to know the extent to which this occurs. A rare recorded example of self-censorship dates from shortly after the anthrax attacks of 2001. Harold Garner and his research team discovered that a unique genetic "barcode" could be inserted into laboratory-held strains of deadly pathogens, thus potentially enabling forensic investigators to track a biological weapon back to its source. A description of this discovery was also, according to Garner, "information that might be misused, to figure out how to evade detection." So his team did not seek to publish it. Instead, they "wrote up a white paper for some of the government agencies, but didn't distribute it widely."[54] In other circumstances, according to Seumas Miller and Michael Selgelid, a "prudent" approach to the dissemination of research findings on a pathogenic microorganism might be to delay it "at least until such time as a vaccine or treatment for the microbe was developed and made widely available."[55] Such an approach was taken in 2013 by scientists working for the California Department of Public Health in a laboratory that diagnoses infant botulism. After discovering a new strain of botulinum toxin that could not be neutralized by any of the available treatments, the scientists consulted with government officials and colleagues and later submitted an incomplete account of their findings to the *Journal of Infectious Diseases*. The article, as published, omitted information on how a reader could manufacture a toxin against which there was no medical defense, and the journal undertook later to publish the complete article once a new treatment had been developed.[56]

In general, however, redaction of text is regarded as antiscientific, as it prevents the replication and testing of experiments. As such it is unlikely to attract favor as an alternative to either full publication or nonpublication. Recent experience shows that journal editors tend to resist the idea of publishing anything less than a full account of research, and in so doing they tend to refer to public health imperatives. For example, *Nature* editor Philip Campbell argued in 2011 "It is essential for public health that the full details of any scientific analysis of flu viruses be available to researchers."[57] He was responding to the NSABB's initial recommendation that redacted versions of Fouchier's and Kawaoka's H5N1 papers be published; the response of *Science* editor Bruce Alberts was similar:

> *Science* has concerns about withholding potentially important public-health information from responsible influenza researchers. Many scientists within the influenza community have a bona fide need to know the details of this research in order to protect the public, especially if they currently are working with related strains of the virus. . . . Our response will be heavily dependent upon the further steps taken by the U.S. government to set forth a written, transparent plan to ensure that any information that is omitted from the publication will be provided to all those responsible scientists who request it, as part of their legitimate efforts to improve public health and safety.[58]

Consistent with these statements, and on the basis of a survey of 127 journal editors in twenty-seven countries, Daniel Patrone and his colleagues predicted, "editors will be reluctant to withhold publication of dual-use research without at least having practical mechanisms for identifying responsible researchers and organizations with legitimate needs for the information and for distributing the information to them."[59] One such mechanism suggested here is "discreet dissemination," which would involve limiting the number of recipients of dual-use research findings rather than limiting the degree to which those findings were described.

If findings could be disseminated directly to those "scientists within the influenza community [who] have a bona fide need" for them, the public health concerns expressed by journal editors would arguably be satisfied. According to Fouchier, he could have shared his virus-mutation findings with "well over 100 organizations around the globe, and probably 1,000 experts."[60] But this claim raises a question: Why, then, should his technology have been transferred also to the hundreds of thousands of people worldwide who read *Science*? One answer, suggested by a US academic who commented on the Fouchier case, is that "fully disseminated research findings" are "the sole coin of the realm for scientists" and are "necessary for university appointments and advancement."[61] An alternative would be instead to subordinate, in certain circumstances, the career interests of individual scientists to the interests of public health and national security. In doing this, though, it would be important for a government not only to be satisfied with the scientific soundness of dual-use research but also to avoid international accusations of excessive secrecy in a matter it deems to be of biological weapons concern. Accordingly, the necessary characteristics of "discreet dissemination" as a biosecurity practice would be

- All direct financial costs of dissemination are borne by the government of the country where the research findings originate
- The government arranges dissemination of the research findings to other researchers, in full accordance with a list of names and work addresses supplied by the authors of the findings
- Findings so disseminated are accompanied by a statement by the editor of a scientific journal indicating that reviewers are satisfied with the scientific quality of the research; and
- The findings are simultaneously disseminated, via the United Nations Office at Geneva, to all BWC member states

Even if "discreet dissemination" could offer a way out of the secure or stifle dilemma arising from dual-use pathogen research, eventually that dilemma itself could be overtaken by another once a dreaded disease outbreak was under way. This third kind of biosecurity dilemma (the subject of part III) potentially arises when a government's concern for national security shapes the response to rather than the prevention of an outbreak. The challenge at that point is to respond to the spread of disease in a way that is robust enough to be effective but not so much as to be counterproductive. This is the "remedy or overkill" dilemma.

NOTES

1. United Nations Office at Geneva, "Convention on the Prohibition of the Development, Production and Stockpiling of Bacteriological (Biological) and Toxin Weapons and on Their Destruction," April 10, 1972, http://www.unog .ch/80256EDD006B8954/%28httpAssets%29/C4048678A93B6934C1257188 004848D0/$file/BWC-text-English.pdf.
2. United Nations Office at Geneva, "Final Document of the Seventh Review Conference," Report No. BWC/CONF.VII/7 (January 13, 2012), http://www .unog.ch/80256EDD006B8954/%28httpAssets%29/3E2A1AA4CF86184BC 1257D960032AA4E/$file/BWC_CONF.VII_07+%28E%29.pdf, 16.
3. Gunnar Jeremias and Jan van Aken, "Harnessing Global Trade Data for Biological Arms Control," *Nonproliferation Review* 13, no. 2 (2006): 204.
4. Australia Group, "Guidelines for Transfers of Sensitive Chemical or Biological Items," June 2012, http://www.australiagroup.net/en/guidelines.html.
5. Australia Group, "Control List of Dual-use Biological Equipment and Related Technology and Software," January 2014, http://www.australiagroup.net/en/dual _biological.html.
6. Australia Group, "New Measures to Fight the Spread of Chemical and Biological Weapons," June 2002, http://www.australiagroup.net/en/agm_june2002.html.
7. ComLaw, Australian government, "Defence Trade Controls Act 2012," 2012, http://www.comlaw.gov.au/Details/C2012A00153, sec. 10.
8. Ibid., sec. 11.4.
9. Australian Department of Defence, "The Defence and Strategic Goods List," n.d., http://www.defence.gov.au/deco/DSGL.asp (accessed October 19, 2015).
10. Australian Department of Defence, "Regulation Impact Statement: Defence Trade Controls Bill 2011," October 2011, http://ris.finance.gov.au/files/2011/11/03 -Defence-Export-Controls-RIS.pdf.
11. Leigh Dayton, "Australian Researchers Rattled by Export Control Law," *Science* 339 (March 15, 2013): 1263.
12. EUR-Lex, "Council Regulation (EC) No. 428/2009 of May 5, 2009: Setting Up a Community Regime for the Control of Exports, Transfer, Brokering and Transit of Dual-Use Items," http://eur-lex.europa.eu/LexUriServ/LexUriServ.do?uri=OJ:L:200 9:134:0001:0269:en:PDF, article 2.2.
13. Ibid., annex 1.
14. Ronald J. Jackson et al., "Expression of Mouse Interleukin-4 by a Recombinant Ectromelia Virus Suppresses Cytolytic Lymphocyte Responses and Overcomes Genetic Resistance to Mousepox," *Journal of Virology* 75, no. 3 (2001): 1205–10.

15. William J. Broad, "Australians Create a Deadly Mouse Virus," *New York Times*, January 23, 2001, http://www.nytimes.com/2001/01/23/health/23MOUS.html.

16. Ibid.

17. Rachel Nowak, "Killer Mousepox Virus Raises Bioterror Fears," *New Scientist*, January 10, 2001, http://www.newscientist.com/article/dn311-killer-mousepox-virus -raises-bioterror-fears.html#.U5bAoCjyQ3l.

18. Jeronimo Cello, Aniko V. Paul, and Eckard Wimmer, "Chemical Synthesis of Poliovirus cDNA: Generation of Infectious Virus in the Absence of Natural Template," *Science* 297 (August 9, 2002): 1016–18.

19. Joby Warrick, "Custom-Built Pathogens Raise Bioterror Fears," *Washington Post*, July 31, 2006, A01.

20. Jennifer Couzin, "A Call for Restraint on Biological Data," *Science* 297 (August 2, 2002): 749.

21. Donald Kennedy, "A Not-So-Cheap Stunt (Response)," *Science* 297 (August 2, 2002): 770.

22. "Statement on the Consideration of Biodefence and Biosecurity," *Nature* 421 (February 20, 2003): 771.

23. US Department of Health and Human Services, "HHS Will Lead Government-Wide Efforts to Enhance Biosecurity in 'Dual Use' Research," March 4, 2004, http://osp.od.nih.gov/announcement/thu-2004-03-04-0000/hhs-announcement -march-2004-re-establishing-nsabb.

24. Jon Cohen, "HHS Asks PNAS to Pull Bioterrorism Paper," *Science* 308 (June 3, 2005): 1395.

25. Scott Shane, "Paper Describes Potential Poisoning of Milk," *New York Times*, June 29, 2005, A20.

26. Lawrence M. Wein and Yifan Liu, "Analyzing a Bioterror Attack on the Food Supply: The Case of Botulinum Toxin in Milk," *Proceedings of the National Academy of Sciences* 102, no. 28 (2005): 9984–89.

27. Bruce Alberts, "Modelling Attacks on the Food Supply," *Proceedings of the National Academy of Sciences* 102, no. 28 (2005): 9737.

28. Jeffery K. Taubenberger et al., "Characterization of the 1918 Influenza Virus Polymerase Genes," *Nature* 437 (October 6, 2005): 889–93; Terrence M. Tumpey et al., "Characterization of the Reconstructed 1918 Spanish Influenza Pandemic Virus," *Science* 310 (October 7, 2005): 77–80

29. Ray Kurzweil and Bill Joy, "Recipe for Destruction," *New York Times*, October 17, 2005, http://www.nytimes.com/2005/10/17/opinion/recipe-for-destruction.html.

30. Jocelyn Kaiser, "Resurrected Influenza Virus Yields Secrets of Deadly 1918 Pandemic," *Science* 310 (October 7, 2005): 29.

31. Andreas von Bubnoff, "The 1918 Flu Virus Is Resurrected," *Nature* 437 (October 6, 2005): 795.

32. Denise Grady and William J. Broad, "Journals Asked to Cut Details of Flu Studies," *New York Times*, December 21, 2011, A1.

33. National Institutes of Health, "National Science Advisory Board for Biosecurity Findings and Recommendations, March 29–30, 2012," https://www.nih.gov/sites /default/files/about-nih/nih-director/statements/collins/03302012_NSABB _Recommendations.pdf.

34. Martin Enserink, "Will Dutch Allow 'Export' of Controversial Flu Study?," *Science* 336 (April 20, 2012): 285.
35. Martin Enserink, "Dutch Government OK's Publication of H5N1 Study," *Science* website, April 27, 2012, http://news.sciencemag.org/2012/04/dutch -government-oks-publication-h5n1-study.
36. EUR-Lex, "Council Regulation (EC) No. 428/2009, annex 1.
37. Sander Herfst et al., "Airborne Transmission of Influenza A/H5N1 Virus between Ferrets," *Science* 336 (June 22, 2012): 1534.
38. Robert Roos, "Experts Call for Alternatives to 'Gain-of-Function' Flu Studies," CIDRAP News, University of Minnesota, May 22, 2014, http://www.cidrap.umn .edu/news-perspective/2014/05/experts-call-alternatives-gain-function-flu-studies.
39. Martin Enserink, "Flu Researcher Ron Fouchier Loses Legal Fight Over H5N1 Studies," *Science*, September 25, 2013, http://news.sciencemag.org/health/2013/09 /flu-researcher-ron-fouchier-loses-legal-fight-over-h5n1-studies.
40. Martin Enserink, "Dutch Appeals Court Dodges Decision on Hotly Debated H5N1 Papers," *Science* website, July 16, 2015, http://news.sciencemag.org/europe/2015/07 /dutch-appeals-court-dodges-decision-hotly-debated-h5n1-papers.
41. "Permissible Medical Experiments," in *Trials of War Criminals before the Nuremberg Military Tribunals under Control Council Law* 10, vol. 2 (Washington, DC: US Government Printing Office, 1949), 181–82.
42. International Committee of the Red Cross, "Preventing Hostile Use of the Life Sciences: From Ethics and Law to Best Practice," November 11, 2004, https://www.icrc .org/eng/resources/documents/misc/biotechnology-principles-of-practice-111104.htm.
43. World Health Organization, "Technical Consultation on H5N1 Research Issues: Consensus Points," February 2012, http://www.who.int/influenza/human_animal _interface/consensus_points/en/.
44. National Institutes of Health, "National Science Advisory Board for Biosecurity Findings and Recommendations," March 29–30, 2012, https://www.nih.gov/sites /default/files/about-nih/nih-director/statements/collins/03302012_NSABB _Recommendations.pdf.
45. Andrew Fowler, "Building the Perfect Bug," *Foreign Correspondent*, ABC Television (Australia), March 13, 2012, http://www.abc.net.au/foreign/content/2012 /s3452543.htm.
46. National Institutes of Health, "National Science Advisory Board."
47. Steve Connor, "No Way of Stopping Leak of Deadly New Flu, Says Terror Chief," *Independent* (London), February 8, 2012, http://www.independent.co.uk/news /science/no-way-of-stopping-leak-of-deadly-new-flu-says-terror-chief-6660997.html.
48. National Institutes of Health, "National Science Advisory Board."
49. World Health Organization, "Cumulative Number of Confirmed Human Cases of Avian Influenza A(H5N1) Reported to WHO," October 15, 2015, http://www .who.int/influenza/human_animal_interface/H5N1_cumulative_table_archives/en/.
50. Herfst et al., "Airborne Transmission," 1534.
51. Michael J. Selgelid and Lorna Weir, "Reflections on the Synthetic Production of Poliovirus," *Bulletin of the Atomic Scientists* 66, no. 3 (2010): 6.
52. Yoshihiro Kawaoka, "H5N1: Flu Transmission Work Is Urgent," *Nature* 482 (February 9, 2012): 155.

53. Sonia Ben Ouagrham-Gormley, "Barriers to Bioweapons: Intangible Obstacles to Proliferation," *International Security* 36, no. 4 (2012): 112–13.
54. David Malakoff, "Hey, You've Got to Hide Your Work Away," *Science* 342 (October 4, 2013): 71.
55. Seumas Miller and Michael J. Selgelid, *Ethical and Philosophical Consideration of the Dual-Use Dilemma in the Biological Sciences* (New York: Springer, 2008), 45.
56. Nell Greenfieldboyce, "Why Scientists Held Back Details on a Unique Botulinum Toxin," NPR News, October 9, 2013, http://www.npr.org/blogs/health /2013/10/11/230957188/why-scientists-held-back-details-on-a-unique-botulinum -toxin; Nir Dover et al., "Molecular Characterization of a Novel Botulinum Neurotoxin Type H Gene," *Journal of Infectious Diseases* 209, no. 2 (2014): 192–202.
57. "Bird Flu: Research Row as US Raises Terror Fears," BBC News, December 21, 2011, http://www.bbc.co.uk/news/world-us-canada-16279365.
58. Kathy Wren, "Science: Editor-in-Chief Bruce Alberts on Publication of H5N1 Avian Influenza Research," American Association for the Advancement of Science, December 20, 2011, http://www.aaas.org/news/science-editor-chief-bruce -alberts-publication-h5n1-avian-influenza-research.
59. Daniel Patrone, David Resnik, and Lisa Chin, "Biosecurity and the Review and Publication of Dual-Use Research of Concern," *Biosecurity and Bioterrorism* 10, no. 3 (2012): 292.
60. Doreen Carvajal, "Scientist in Bird Flu Study Says He Is Not Convinced Censorship Is a Safeguard," *New York Times*, December 22, 2011, A28.
61. Abraham R. Liboff, "Sunday Dialogue: Bird Flu Experiments," *New York Times*, January 29, 2012, SR2.

PART III
REMEDY OR OVERKILL

5

SOCIAL DISTANCING AND NATIONAL SECURITY

IN LATE 2011, when a journalist asked Ron Fouchier about the possibility of terrorism involving a laboratory-created influenza virus, the virologist remarked, "Nature is the biggest bioterrorist."[1] In seeking thus to downplay the threat posed by *scientist*-bioterrorists, Fouchier also conflated that threat with the risk of naturally occurring infectious disease outbreaks. From a disease-control perspective, such conflation makes sense because many of the basic measures needed to protect populations against natural outbreaks are essentially the same as would be required to mitigate the effects of a biological attack. For this reason, in 2002 the 55th World Health Assembly (WHA) passed a resolution stating that "one of the most effective methods of preparing for deliberately caused disease is to strengthen public health surveillance and response activities for naturally or accidentally occurring diseases."[2] It is possible that, eventually, the *preventive* biosecurity practices discussed in part II of this book will fail, so it is necessary for governments to have a good capacity for responding to actualized biosecurity risks. Even if biological attacks were to not occur, a disease outbreak of natural origin may attract concern from a national security perspective.

Regardless of its origin, once a dreaded disease outbreak is under way, public health responses generally fall into two categories: pharmaceutical and nonpharmaceutical. Much of the discussion thus far has been focused on the prospect of laboratory-based pathogen research leading to the development of new and better drugs and vaccines. A problem with relying on pharmaceutical defenses, however, is that individuals and governments might find that these cannot be deployed when needed or in the quantities required to mitigate and contain a disease outbreak. In the event of an influenza pandemic, for example, antiviral medication to treat infection and prevent its spread could be in short supply, and a vaccine matched to the pandemic virus would not be available until several months after the pandemic virus started to circulate. In the meantime, while the imperative to save lives remained strong, nonpharmaceutical responses to an outbreak might be the only kind available. Accordingly, the next part of the discussion of biosecurity dilemmas shifts to the advantages and disadvantages of implementing "social distancing"—a nonpharmaceutical disease-control measure that involves the physical separation of healthy and (potentially) unhealthy people for the sake of public health and national security. Consideration of the "remedy or overkill" dilemma is then continued in chapter 6 to cover the distancing to be achieved by international border controls and travel restrictions.

In the context of a naturally occurring infectious disease outbreak, the remedy or overkill dilemma is one that potentially arises when a government chooses to frame a health problem as being also a security problem. On the one hand, ascribing security status to a disease outbreak might be a beneficial move to garner additional resources, effort, and powers for protecting the health of populations within and across nations. On the other hand, disease-control practices driven by a supposed security imperative might be harmful; that is, so heavy-handed as to be counterproductive to public health or excessively injurious to national economies and human rights. Social distancing, like the practice of "bordering" (or managing borders), is conducive to being motivated by security concerns. So resorting to both kinds of practice in response to disease contagion necessarily involves curtailing individuals' freedom of movement. As such, the discussion incorporates ideas about public health ethics as well as security policy. The remedy or overkill dilemma is explored by reference to two dreaded diseases: drug-resistant TB and Ebola. In each case, pharmaceutical-based responses tend to be unavailable, and there is an ethical concern that any move to "securitize" the disease should support rather than undermine the protection of public health.

DISEASE OUTBREAKS, SECURITY, AND ETHICS

How might a naturally occurring infectious disease outbreak be reckoned an issue of national security? One possible answer is that a disease's "security-ness" emerges when its effects reach or approach "the point of imposing an intolerable burden on society."[3] Direct effects include the quantum of illness and death; indirect effects include the social disruption and debilitation caused by popular dread of the disease. The latter are of particular concern for present purposes because dread can be a powerful political commodity and because the security status of a disease outbreak can be a matter of political judgment. As discussed earlier, dread can be engendered or exacerbated by such factors as the unfamiliarity of an infectious disease, the speed with which it spreads, or any apparent lack of a pharmaceutical remedy. When the state is the referent object of security, and when dread of a disease undermines the ability of the state to function, it becomes empirically and politically plausible to characterize that disease in terms of national security. Partly this is because such characterization accords with individual citizens' own *sense* of insecurity. Fear of contagion compromises the day-to-day human interaction that sustains society, and societies function and survive largely because people have regular contact with and depend on each other. During an outbreak of a deadly disease, as Marcel Verweij and Angus Dawson have argued, "routine activities become the focus of concerns about potential modes of disease transmission, and in the face of dramatic risks this is likely to affect everyone's attitudes to strangers, friends and to themselves."[4] Moreover, as Andrew Price-Smith has observed, the fearsome and disruptive influence of a disease outbreak can eventually undermine the power and internal cohesion of a state.[5]

An early example of the relationship between disease, dread, and societal collapse is found in Thucydides's *History of the Peloponnesian War*. The Athenian general, who survived the plague in fifth-century BCE Athens, wrote:

> Athens owed to the plague the beginnings of a state of unprecedented lawlessness. . . . No fear of god or law of man had a restraining influence. As for the gods, it seemed to be the same thing whether one worshipped them or not, when one saw the good and the bad dying indiscriminately. As for offences against human law, no one expected to live long enough to be brought to trial and punished.[6]

This scenario is no different in its essentials from our more recent experiences of fearsome diseases and fearful populations. In 1994, for example, when cases of plague were reported in the Indian city of Surat, hundreds of thousands of people fled the city in a single night.[7] In 2003, during the SARS outbreak, in some parts of China riots erupted following rumors of government plans to establish patient isolation wards.[8] Such incidents demonstrate both the panic created when populations imagine a disease spreading out of control and the fragility of the social contract under which citizens place trust in their government to protect them in times of crisis.

In the aftermath of the SARS outbreak, the emergence of the highly pathogenic H5N1 bird flu virus in late 2003 served to compound political concerns about the disruptive and demoralizing effects of a deadly and contagious disease. The mutation of this virus into a pandemic form was a fearsome prospect because it could result in a disease outbreak causing illness and death on a large scale, over a wide area, in a short space of time. A 2006 pandemic preparedness plan drafted by the US president's Homeland Security Council stated that "the impact of a severe [influenza] pandemic may be . . . comparable to that of war."[9] The plan warned:

> Absenteeism across multiple sectors related to personal illness, illness in family members, fear of contagion, or public health measures to limit contact with others could threaten the functioning of critical infrastructure, the movement of goods and services, and operation of institutions such as schools and universities. A pandemic would thus have significant implications for the economy, national security, and the basic functioning of society.[10]

Accordingly, the council adopted the position that a "necessary enabler of pandemic preparedness" was that this be viewed "as a national security issue."[11] In essence, it was a move to "securitize" pandemic influenza so that this dreaded disease risk might be better resisted.

In their 1998 book *Security: A New Framework for Analysis*, Barry Buzan and his coauthors theorized on the political process by which an issue acquires security status (securitization). They argued that "security issues" are distinguished from "the normal run of the merely political," and that, to "count" as the former, "threats and vulnerabilities" must be "staged as existential threats to a referent object by a securitizing actor who thereby generates endorsement of emergency measures beyond rules that would otherwise bind."[12] Although their book did not address issues arising in the sphere of health policy, a number of other works have since drawn on securitization theory to explain, assess, or contest the security significance of naturally occurring infectious disease outbreaks.[13] In addition, some historical accounts of government responses to disease outbreaks presaged the emphasis in securitization theory on the extreme nature of threats and the extraordinary nature of responses.[14] For example, in a 1992 essay on perceptions of plague in colonial India in the late nineteenth century, Rajnarayan Chandavarkar wrote:

> The plague represented the apotheosis of the threat of disease. . . . Immediate and summary action now seemed imperative. Policy initiatives which had once seemed impolitic now seemed indispensable; those which seemed to lie beyond the capacity of the state suddenly fell within its grasp and no effort or expense was to be spared. Intervention in a style which was considered unthinkable before was now seriously pursued.[15]

This account resonates strongly with the notion that securitization involves the transgressing of social rules, norms, and settled expectations that would otherwise bind governments and their people. In general, such transgression tends to be matched to the urgency of the situation. That is, claims about the security status of an issue are often invoked, and other (nonsecurity) interests are subordinated because time is of the essence and the pursuit of some greater good must happen quickly.

Acting in emergency mode can be risky, however, and any temporary subordination of supposedly lesser goods (such as individual freedom) might in fact be counterproductive when pursuing a security objective. Relevant to this point, Chandavarkar's account of plague in India also described how the aggressive intrusion by British authorities into people's private lives occasioned "a general refusal of state intervention."[16] For the inhabitants of Bombay, for example, it was "preferable by far to flee the city . . . than to place their trust in a government which . . . now intervened in an arbitrary and brutal manner."[17] The lesson to be drawn from this and similar experiences is that, although political claims about the security status of a particular disease outbreak might refer to the importance of a swift and aggressive response, haste and zeal can sometimes undermine rather than support disease-control objectives. The concern is that emergency measures, once implemented, could impinge on the interests of the people to be protected to such an extent that the securitization of a disease becomes illegitimate.

Buzan and his coauthors argue that "avoiding excessive and irrational securitization is . . . a legitimate social, political and economic objective of considerable importance."[18] Thus they incorporate the beginnings of a normative dimension into a theory that is otherwise merely descriptive of a political process. For present purposes, the normative concern is that securitization in the sphere of contemporary health policy (if it is warranted at all) should, over time, protect rather than endanger public health. It is a concern first raised by Stefan Elbe in a 2006 article that opened up a normative debate on HIV/AIDS and security. Elbe acknowledged that the securitization of HIV/AIDS "could accrue vital economic, social, and political benefits for millions of affected people by raising awareness of the pandemic's debilitating global consequences and by bolstering resources for international AIDS initiatives."[19] However, he also warned of the risk that

framing the issue as a security issue pushes responses to the disease away from civil society toward the much less transparent workings of military and intelligence organizations, which also possess the power to override human rights and civil liberties—including those of persons living with HIV/AIDS.[20]

Observing instances of such people being "ostracized and even persecuted by some states for their illness," Elbe argued that framing HIV/AIDS as a national security threat risks fueling "exclusionary and dehumanizing responses."[21] Indeed, one such response was proposed in 2008 by legislators in Indonesia's Papua Province: HIV/AIDS patients being required to have a microchip implanted beneath the skin. Patients deemed "sexually aggressive" would thus be more easily identified, tracked, and punished were they to infect others with HIV. One of the proponents explained at the time: "The health situation is extraordinary, so we have to take extraordinary action."[22]

From a public health perspective, the problem with treating infected people in this way is that it might cause them to avoid engaging with a government's disease-control efforts. As a result, and especially if the disease is contagious, the health situation of those people and public health conditions in general are made worse. Ethically speaking, it is a problem with the balance of consequences: an emergency measure causing more harm than benefit. An idea worth considering, then, is that securitization should be ethically sound. That is, governments should pursue positive rather than negative securitization when confronting a serious disease outbreak. Rita Floyd, in offering a consequentialist evaluation of security, has defined "a positive securitization" as "an intense political solution that within the margins of moral rightness, and preferably based upon the political interest of the majority, benefits a security problem."[23] Negative securitization, by contrast, is "an intense political solution that benefits the few; and/or with a too narrow focus to address the underlying problems of the prevailing insecurity."[24] Floyd's is clearly a utilitarian ethics of security, according to which the maximization of good consequences is pursued. As such, there is a connection here with the utilitarianism that dominates thinking about the ethics of public health.[25] Just as the personal security of individual human beings is often rendered secondary to the security of "human collectivities," so too do public health ethics tend to emphasize the collective interests of entire populations.[26]

When it comes to contagious diseases, the need for applying ethical principles is relatively unfamiliar, especially in more developed parts of the world. This is largely due to the fact that modern bioethics has focused overwhelmingly on health as experienced at the individual level rather than the broad population level. In Europe and North America in the late nineteenth and early twentieth centuries, improvements in sanitation and hygiene served to reduce the incidence of illness and death caused by infectious microorganisms. From the mid-twentieth century on, the widespread availability of antibiotics and vaccines further diminished the magnitude of infectious diseases as a public health problem. This created an opportunity, in the West at least, to protect human health against the now-greater problem of noncommunicable diseases, with the sufferers treated on a more individualized basis. In turn, the reduced need to address people's common vulnerability to contagion occasioned a shift in ethical emphasis away from public interests and toward private interests.[27] Today this is reflected most strongly in the high degree of attention bioethicists devote to the principle of individual autonomy. When it comes to such matters as informed consent to treatment for a noncommunicable disease like cancer, affording moral primacy to patients' individual rights and interests is generally regarded as appropriate. However, when a deadly disease is contagious and a pharmaceutical solution is unavailable, such emphasis is harder to maintain and justify. Effective disease control might rather seem to require imposing limits on the exercise of individual freedom.

In the contemplation of social distancing (placing limits on people's freedom of movement and association) as a nonpharmaceutical response to an outbreak, the critical consideration is that a person infected with a contagious disease is both *at* risk (from the disease) and *a* risk (to others). In one sense that person is a disease vector from whom the broader population should be protected (an immediate greater good). In another sense, though, he or she is a disease victim possessing human rights whose health and well-being should be protected (an immediate individual good).[28] A policy dilemma arises over the relative impor-tance of achieving each immediate good, and it is compounded by the notion that two long-term greater goods are also at stake: public confidence in the protective capacity of public health and healthcare systems and public confidence in the protection of individual rights. Regarding the latter, it is nevertheless important to acknowledge that rights protected by law are not (as a matter of law) protected always or absolutely. In some international human rights treaties, for example, there are long-standing provisions that allow governments to curtail or suspend citizens' rights for a variety of purposes, including public health. Although mea-sures to control an infectious disease might impinge on an individual's freedom, these would not necessarily constitute an *illegal* infringement. This is best illus-trated by the 1984 Siracusa Principles on the Limitation and Derogation Pro-visions, which were amended to the 1966 International Covenant on Civil and Political Rights. The principles provide that

> Public health may be invoked as a ground for limiting certain rights in order to allow a state to take measures dealing with a serious threat to the health of the population or individual members of the population. These measures must be specifically aimed at preventing disease or injury or providing care for the sick and injured.[29]

The wording of this legal provision reflects a number of ethical principles that are applicable to public health policy relevant to determining whether positive or negative securitization of a disease outbreak is occurring. The most important principle, arguably, is that the permissibility of a rights-limiting measure depends on its effectiveness. Limitation is justified if a given disease-control measure is effective in dealing with a health risk. If it is not, and if it causes harm instead, then limiting freedom of movement, for example, is unethical. Other principles identified by various authors include necessity of harm avoidance (of clear and measurable harm to people if specific disease-control measures are not implemented), proportionality (the least intrusive and burdensome disease-control measure should be implemented), reciprocity (society should support the curtailing of individual liberties in the discharge of that obligation only if individuals agree), and nondiscrimination (the curtailing of rights should not be experienced by anyone on the basis of membership in a particular group).[30]

The "extremely difficult ethical question" highlighted by Michael Selgelid is knowing "how to strike a balance between the utilitarian aim of promoting public health, on the one hand, and libertarian aims of protecting privacy and freedom of movement, on the other."[31] The task of appropriately balancing and simultaneously pursuing these two sets of interests is made even more difficult (and more important) with the insertion of a security element. In particular, the dread factor that is so often present in anything to do with "security" can have a distorting effect on policy and practice. Some ethicists have argued that the powerful ability of some infectious diseases to engender fear often leads to "rapid, emotionally driven decision making about the care of individual patients and about public health policies" even when these decisions "challenge generally accepted medical ethics principles."[32] At the intersection of public health, security, and ethics, therefore, the challenge for government officials is to securitize a disease outbreak in a positive way. This is a challenge of particular gravity when confronting dreaded diseases against which pharmaceutical resources cannot be used. Accordingly, the next section focuses on nonpharmaceutical responses to drug-resistant TB and Ebola.

SOCIAL DISTANCING AS A BIOSECURITY PRACTICE

In the absence of vaccines or therapeutic drugs, when confronting the spread of a dreaded disease the decision may be made to prevent or slow contagion by distancing people from each other. In this chapter, the discussion of social distancing as a biosecurity practice focuses on isolation and quarantine. Both of these centuries-old disease-control measures are conducive to being motivated by security concerns, and both infringe (for better or for worse) on individuals' freedom of movement. Isolation involves separating people known to be infected with a contagious disease from healthy people; quarantine involves restricting the movement of healthy people who (might) have been exposed to a contagious disease. In both cases the duration of a person's experience of social distancing should be commensurate only with the period during which transmission of the relevant microorganism to another person is possible.

Until 2003 it had been many decades since the use of isolation and quarantine had occurred regularly or on a large scale anywhere in the world. Thus, when these measures were implemented in response to SARS (a disease then unknown to medical science), the measures were unfamiliar and at times alarming to local populations. In China, for example, the SARS outbreak and the government's response to it were associated with widespread civil unrest and subsequent damage to property. Communities set up blockades to deter outsiders from entering certain areas out of fear that they carried the disease, and on several occasions mobs attacked and burned quarantine centers that local authorities had established in their villages.[33] This experience of confronting a deadly contagion, though unfamiliar in the early twenty-first century, is nevertheless directly comparable to historical circumstances in which only nonpharmaceutical measures were available to control a disease. Moreover, the reaction to SARS is a warning of the need to ensure disease-control efforts are not stymied by panic. This is important from a security perspective because, as Buzan and his coauthors have argued, security politics sometimes manifests as "panic politics."[34] Dreaded diseases are more likely to be framed and addressed in security terms, and the ethical concern that arises then is that emergency disease-control measures should not be ineffective, counterproductive, or unjust (negative securitization).

Drug-Resistant TB and Long-Term Isolation[35]

Illness caused by drug-resistant *Mycobacterium tuberculosis* bacteria (transmissible via airborne droplets) is a fearsome prospect. Infection is harder to survive and more difficult to treat successfully than ordinary TB illness. The bacteria can build up resistance to anti-TB drugs if treatment is inadequate, and bacteria that are resistant to first-line drugs cause multidrug-resistant (MDR) TB. It is then only possible to treat an infected person with stronger second-line drugs administered over a longer period of time. However, if this treatment too is inadequate, the targeted bacteria can mutate further into a form against which almost no drug is effective: extensively drug-resistant (XDR) TB. In its 2014 Global Tuberculosis Report, the WHO estimated that 480,000 people worldwide developed MDR-TB in 2013 and that 9 percent of those (more than 43,000 people) had XDR-TB.[36] The significance is that, as drug-resistance becomes more widespread, a pharmaceutical and *bacteria*-centric response to all forms of TB moves further out of reach. In turn, the relative importance of disease control centered on the *people* who have TB illness (and who can thus spread it to others) grows. It is in this context that emergency measures have been proposed and implemented.

In 1993, evidence of a resurgence of TB in developed countries and the emergence of drug-resistant strains of *Mycobacterium tuberculosis* prompted the WHO to declare this disease burden "a global emergency."[37] The identification of XDR-TB in South Africa in 2006 then led the WHO to call for "urgent preventative action."[38] The organization's 2007 World Health Report warned, "XDR-TB is as transmissible as its treatable counterparts . . . [so] it is of paramount importance that all tuberculosis infections are identified and treated promptly."[39] Later, the language of security began to surround the disease. For example, in 2008 a member of the security committee of Russia's State Duma declared that TB posed "a real threat" to Russia's security at a time when the country was experiencing a labor shortage.[40] In 2010 the chairman of Ghana's Parliamentary Select Committee on Health argued that TB "must be declared a national security threat," and added that "if this was done [then] TB would be given the attention it deserved by all Ghanaians in fighting it."[41] The available epidemiological data on XDR-TB provide a basis for making plausible claims about its security status, just as a comparison is made to other infectious diseases that are already being addressed in security terms. For example, compared to HIV, which is not readily transmissible, it is much harder to protect oneself against infection by airborne *Mycobacterium tuberculosis*. And, whereas pandemic influenza also spreads through the air, TB bacteria can be far more deadly than influenza virus, especially if they are drug resistant.

XDR-TB bacteria are virtually unconquerable using antibiotics, so there is a compelling case for placing these microorganisms in an epidemiological "dead end" by preventing the movement of the human host. Indeed, the idea of a TB "emergency" and using social distancing as a nonpharmaceutical response measure might have particular appeal for the governments of countries experiencing a high burden of drug-resistant TB. However, it is worth noting that the experience of TB patients' interests being subordinated to national interest has sometimes been a distressing one. In 2007, for example, thirteen MDR-TB patients in South Africa who had forced their way out of a hospital and demanded to be treated as outpatients were ordered back to their beds by an interim court order. Against the argument of provincial health authorities in favor of forced isolation, the patients claimed (to no avail) that this would result in them losing their jobs and welfare benefits.[42] Following this incident a protest by MDR- and XDR-TB patients at a Johannesburg hospital, who were calling for an end to "prison-like" conditions there, became violent, and one patient was shot.[43] By 2008, when twenty MDR-TB patients being confined at another South African hospital attacked a nurse and security guards, uprisings of this kind were becoming commonplace in that country.[44] Afterward, the doctor in charge of Port Elizabeth's Jose Pearson Hospital, which has guarded gates and a perimeter fence topped with razor wire, told a BBC journalist that forced isolation was the only option: "MDR and XDR, if not controlled, are almost like biological warfare against the population."[45]

Although such dramatic framing of the issue can serve to legitimize strict social distancing as a biosecurity practice, there is also the risk that the perceived severity of those measures might be counterproductive to disease control. Long-term isolation might well be regarded as an effective and inexpensive response to the grave risk posed by drug-resistant TB. However, any immediate good that is achieved is probably outweighed by the long-term harmfulness of such an extreme measure. The horrific prospect of forced isolation works to drive symptomatic TB sufferers underground, away from the attention of clinical caregivers and public health practitioners, because of a "loss of community trust."[46] Inasmuch as those distrustful patients opt for inadequate TB drug treatment through unofficial channels, the result is likely to be an exacerbation of the very conditions that occasioned the development of drug resistance in the first place. One way of mitigating this risk might be to temper a security-oriented approach with a commitment to acting in a way that is ethically sound over the long term. The WHO's ethical advice to governments is to avoid involuntary isolation; it should be "a very last resort" rather than a standard response.[47] But the question then remains: How can *voluntary* isolation be achieved if isolation *per se* is the only way to stop XDR-TB from spreading? If "no effort or expense [is] to be spared," what would it take for someone with TB to consent and keep consenting to long-term isolation?[48]

Perhaps positive securitization of drug-resistant TB could involve the application of the principle of reciprocity: when individuals agree to curtail their freedom out of a sense of social obligation, society in turn supports those individuals in the fulfilment of that obligation.[49] From a support perspective, the problem at present with isolating XDR-TB patients is the frequent difficulty of characterizing them as "patients" in the sense that they are receiving treatment. In wealthier settings, available treatment could be of indefinite duration and indeterminate cost, possibly limited only by an ill person's life expectancy. In underresourced settings, where treatment is simply too expensive to attempt, isolation in a TB hospital is akin to being a virtual prisoner in a hopeless situation. An alternative and more appealing situation would be one in which a patient is able to live in comfortable conditions of confinement and be hopeful of being cured. Bringing about such an arrangement on a large scale would be expensive, to be sure, but the seriousness of XDR-TB as a matter of national security might legitimize the expense. Moreover, the consequent removal of infected people from the general population in a manner not repellent to victims could prove effective over the long term as an exercise in disease control.

In Europe and North America in the nineteenth century, prior to the advent of antibiotics to treat TB, many ill people voluntarily visited a sanatorium in the hope that fresh air, sunlight, and good food would provide a cure. Although from a therapeutic perspective it is not known how effective these visits were, the existence of sanatoria nevertheless facilitated the long-term removal of infectious TB patients from the community.[50] If the idea of again resorting to sanatoria seems strange, it is probably because there is today a settled expectation (in wealthy parts of the world, at least) that pharmaceutical approaches to disease control are sufficient. However, given the risk posed by XDR-TB bacteria and the paucity of drugs available to successfully treat this form of TB illness, there is arguably cause to consider adopting and adapting a measure dating from the pre-antibiotic era. Consistent with the principle of reciprocity, sanatoria for modern-day TB patients would need to offer leading-edge treatment and care (including palliative care) and diagnostic laboratory facilities. They would also need to be a safe, dignified, and comfortable setting—complete with social, educational, and recreational opportunities—where patients undergoing TB treatment (or not, if they so chose) could reside on a long-term basis. In essence, in a twenty-first century TB sanatorium the voluntary surrender of personal liberty would be repaid, and the discharge of a social duty not to infect others would be rewarded, with a government commitment to maximizing the health and lifestyle quality of isolated TB patients.

From the perspective of those inside a sanatorium, further reciprocal measures taken outside would be vitally important as well. First, governments would need to commit to curing sanatorium-based TB patients as quickly as possible so as to minimize the time spent in isolation. Such a commitment could be manifested in urgently sponsoring medical research in the pursuit of more effective antibiotics. Second, people isolated in sanatoria would need to be satisfied that all due effort was under way to achieve universal access to adequate treatment for drug-susceptible TB illness. Otherwise, if the underlying causes of drug resistance were not being addressed, patients' duty-driven isolation would seem to be in vain. Finally, despite the political appeal of isolation as an extraordinary response to XDR-TB, governments would need to inquire sincerely and constantly into the public health benefit of sanatoria. That is, if the liberty of individuals were to be curtailed for years on end, they and their governments would need to be confident that isolation really does achieve a measurable and sufficient benefit for society.[51] Overall, long-term isolation as an emergency measure going "beyond rules that would otherwise bind," could in this way be characterized as positive securitization of XDR-TB.[52]

EBOLA AND GEOGRAPHICAL QUARANTINE

Social distancing as a biosecurity practice can also manifest as negative securitization, and this is one of the lessons to be drawn from the 2014 Ebola outbreak in West Africa. Ebola, like drug-resistant TB, is a dreaded disease and tends not to be susceptible to pharmaceutical countermeasures. The symptoms (high fever, diarrhea, and profuse internal and external bleeding) are horrific, and recorded case-fatality rates have historically been as high as 90 percent. In December 2013 a case of Ebola in rural Guinea sparked the largest-ever outbreak of the disease, an outbreak so vast and so terrifying that it came to be regarded as a threat to national security. When the Ebola virus started spreading, local health officials misdiagnosed the initial cases, so Ebola was not confirmed in Guinea until March 21, 2014.[53] Soon afterward, laboratory tests showed that at least seventy people had died of Ebola, and neighboring Liberia notified the WHO that it had two laboratory-confirmed cases of Ebola.[54] Sierra Leone quickly became the third of three adjoining West African countries within which the Ebola virus mainly proliferated, but small numbers of cases were later also reported in Mali, Nigeria, Senegal, Spain, the United Kingdom, and the United States. In early April 2014 a WHO spokesperson offered the assurance, "The fortunate thing with Ebola is, it's quite difficult to transmit. You have to touch someone. Fortunately for the greater population, the risks are quite small."[55] By late June, however, nearly four hundred people had died during the outbreak, which by then had become the largest ever in terms of cases, deaths, and geographical spread.

On August 8, 2014, WHO director-general Margaret Chan used her authority under the 2005 International Health Regulations (IHRs) to declare the Ebola epidemic to be a "public health emergency of international concern" (PHEIC). Her advice to states with active Ebola transmission (Guinea, Liberia, and Sierra Leone) was to declare a national emergency and activate disaster management plans.[56] A week later the WHO reported that its staff in outbreak zones were seeing "evidence that the numbers of reported cases and deaths vastly underestimate the magnitude of the outbreak," and it warned that "extraordinary measures [are] needed, on a massive scale, to contain the outbreak in settings characterized by extreme poverty, dysfunctional health systems, a severe shortage of doctors, and rampant fear."[57] This fear of Ebola, against the spread of which local authorities appeared helpless, exacerbated social tensions within the affected countries in West Africa that had only recently emerged from years of civil conflict. In turn, a feverish distrust of authority hindered what little disease-control effort could be brought to bear. In late August 2014, for example, riots broke out in the Guinean city of Nzérékoré over rumors that health workers there had deliberately infected people with the Ebola virus.[58] When CDC director Tom Frieden returned to the

United States from a visit to affected countries, he told a media conference on September 2, 2014: "There's . . . a real risk to the stability and security of societies as governments are increasingly challenged to not only control Ebola but provide basic health services, security services, and keep the government running."[59] The Liberian defense minister agreed, telling country representatives on the UN Security Council "Liberia is facing a serious threat to its national existence. The deadly Ebola virus has caused a disruption of the normal functioning of our state."[60] The president of Sierra Leone earlier had remarked, "The very essence of our nation is at stake."[61] Ebola had been framed as a security issue. Unfortunately, though, one particular security-oriented response to this dreaded disease—internal bordering—appeared to be counterproductive to disease control. Within West Africa, as governments approached the outbreak with fearful uncertainty about its future progress, a problem of negative securitization arose in the form of large-scale quarantine zones.

In late July 2014 Sierra Leone's president declared a state of emergency and ordered the quarantine of "all epicenters of the disease" and of "localities and homes where the disease is identified" for a period of sixty to ninety days.[62] Soon afterward, in an operation code-named Octopus, around 750 military personnel deployed to establish and maintain a *cordon sanitaire* (sanitary barrier) based on roadblocks. It was the first instance of geographical quarantine in nearly a century and, in the east of the country where the density of Ebola cases was highest, one area designated as a quarantine zone contained around one million people.[63] A severe downside of large-scale quarantine, however, was that access restrictions pushed up food prices, and this in turn prompted concerns that starvation would pose more of a danger than Ebola itself.[64] In neighboring Liberia, when President Ellen Johnson Sirleaf announced a ninety-day state of emergency in early August, she declared that "extraordinary measures" were required "for the very survival of our state."[65] These measures included military blockades to stop people from Ebola-affected regions in the west of Liberia from entering the capital, Monrovia.[66] More extraordinary still, though, was the sudden imposition and violent enforcement of a *cordon sanitaire* inside the city. On August 20 residents of West Point (a slum area of Monrovia) awoke to find riot police, under orders from President Sirleaf, setting up roadblocks into and out of the area using barbed wire barricades. Amid fears of food shortages among more than sixty thousand people forcibly contained within the quarantine zone, angry crowds clashed with armed soldiers at the barricades, and a local teenager died after being shot.[67] Later, President Sirleaf acknowledged that her decision to quarantine West Point "did not work" and "created more tensions in the society."[68]

By infringing on people's basic and legitimate expectation of freedom of movement the leaders of Sierra Leone and Liberia might have been attempting sincerely to protect the greater part of their citizenry. However, as the West Point example well demonstrates, if disease-control efforts provoke anxiety and violence, they can end up being deleterious both to public health and public safety. Indeed, popular outrage at mass quarantine is understandable given that, in addition to restricting liberty and access to food, this measure "risks placing some individuals who are not infected at a higher risk of becoming infected if groups of people are quarantined together and the disease is transmitted among them."[69] At the same time, it is understandable also that a government might resort to the implementation of nonpharmaceutical disease control when, as was the case during the 2014 Ebola outbreak, vaccines and therapeutic drugs are not available. In the absence of pharmaceutical resources, the governments of Liberia and Sierra Leone tried to block the transmission of a virus simply by blockading the people who might carry it. Nevertheless, doing this was an excessive response to a virus that was known not to spread easily from person to person (e.g., through the air). If geographical quarantine as a biosecurity practice achieved more harm than good, it represented the "overkill" that is negative securitization.

CONCLUSION

When an outbreak of a dreaded disease is under way and a government is inclined to approach it as a matter of national security, a biosecurity dilemma (remedy or overkill) might arise if pharmaceutical approaches are not available. Should authorities use isolation and quarantine as emergency disease-control measures (the "remedy") and thereby run the risk of exacerbating the problem by provoking citizens' refusal to cooperate (the "overkill")? The answer, in some circumstances, might not be obvious. From a public health ethics perspective, there is difficulty enough in satisfying the dual imperative to protect population health as well as individual freedom. Adding a security element compounds the dilemma by raising the stakes. The advantage of appealing to national security might be that urgent action can be taken and resources can be accessed, which would not ordinarily be permissible. The disadvantage, however, might be that securitization of a disease outbreak occasions a repellent heavy-handedness that achieves more harm than help over the long term. In the resorting to social distancing as a biosecurity practice, the critical consideration should be that the disease-control response identifies and helps people who have been exposed to infection. Any response that instead prompts people to conceal themselves or resist help (perhaps violently) is ineffective and, to the extent that the disease is thereby made to spread further, counterproductive.

It is ethically desirable that any move to securitize a dreaded disease should support rather than undermine public health. In the case of XDR-TB, a claim about security status is plausible because the burden of the disease is growing, the bacteria that cause it are transmitted relatively easily, and successful treatment is extremely costly and difficult. The forced isolation of TB patients in settings where they are bereft of hope is a measure that might immediately address a supposed security imperative. Indeed, this action resonates strongly with other security-based arguments calling for the subordination of the rights of the few to the needs of the many. However, forced isolation is also a horrific prospect that is likely to dissuade other patients from engaging with local authorities' disease-control efforts. A better approach to isolation over the long term—positive securitization—might be to expend an extraordinary amount of effort and resources (far more than would ordinarily be politically acceptable) to establish and maintain sanatoria inside which TB patients could enjoy comfort, respect, and hope of a cure.

In the case of Ebola, the 2014 outbreak of that dreaded disease attracted negative securitization. Punctuated by appeals to national security, the response of the Liberian and Sierra Leonean governments was to consign thousands of citizens to the deprivation and danger of a quarantine zone. As a biosecurity practice, the *cordon sanitaire* was a disease-control instrument as blunt in principle as it was sometimes brutal in practice. Nevertheless, the perceived need to use geographical quarantine as an emergency measure is attributable in part to the unavailability of a pharmaceutical-based response to the Ebola virus. In addition, the desperation of decision makers in the worst-affected areas of West Africa was probably occasioned by a prolonged shortage of medical assistance coming from countries elsewhere. As the outbreak progressed, the WHO argued persistently that the better approach to providing Ebola relief was to insert a large number of capable, adequately supplied medical personnel into the situation to treat illness and prevent infection. Such an approach was stymied, however, by externally imposed prohibitions on travel to and from the worst-affected countries. This securing of international borders against transnational contagion, to be discussed in the next chapter, is another biosecurity practice that can give rise to a remedy or overkill dilemma.

NOTES

1. Doreen Carvajal, "Scientist in Bird Flu Study Says He Is Not Convinced Censorship Is a Safeguard," *New York Times*, December 22, 2011, A28.
2. World Health Organization, "Global Public Health Response to Natural Occurrence, Accidental Release or Deliberate Use of Biological and Chemical Agents or

Radionuclear Material that Affect Health," World Health Assembly Resolution No. WHA55.16, May 18, 2002, http://apps.who.int/gb/archive/pdf_files/WHA55/ewha5516.pdf.

3. Christian Enemark, *Disease and Security: Natural Plagues and Biological Weapons in East Asia* (Abingdon, UK: Routledge, 2007), 1.

4. Marcel Verweij and Angus Dawson, "Shutting Up Infected Houses: Infectious Disease Control, Past and Present," *Public Health Ethics* 3, no. 1 (2010): 1.

5. Andrew T. Price-Smith, *Contagion and Chaos: Disease, Ecology, and National Security in the Era of Globalization* (Cambridge, MA: MIT Press, 2009), 2.

6. Thucydides, *History of the Peloponnesian War*, trans. Rex Warner (Harmondsworth, UK: Penguin, 1954), 155.

7. V. Ramalingaswarmi, "Psychosocial Effects of the 1994 Plague Outbreak in Surat, India," *Military Medicine* 166, supplement 2 (2001): 29.

8. Erik Eckholm, "SARS Is the Spark for a Riot in China," *New York Times*, April 29, 2003, A1.

9. US Homeland Security Council, *Implementation Plan for the National Strategy for Pandemic Influenza* (Washington, DC: Homeland Security Council, 2006), 2.

10. Ibid., 1.

11. Ibid., 18.

12. Barry Buzan, Ole Waever, and Jaap de Wilde, *Security: A New Framework for Analysis* (Boulder, CO: Lynne Rienner, 1998), 5.

13. See, for example, Colin McInnes and Kelley Lee, "Health, Security, and Foreign Policy," *Review of International Studies* 32, no. 1 (2006): 5–23; Sara E. Davies, "Securitizing Infectious Disease," *International Affairs* 84, no. 2 (2008): 295–313; Christian Enemark, "Is Pandemic Flu a Security Threat?," *Survival* 51, no. 1 (2009): 191–214; and Simon Rushton, "Global Health Security: Security for Whom? Security from What?," *Political Studies* 59, no. 4 (2011): 779–96.

14. See Price-Smith, *Contagion and Chaos*.

15. Rajnarayan Chandavarkar, "Plague Panic and Epidemic Politics in India, 1896–1914," in *Epidemics and Ideas: Essays on the Historical Perception of Pestilence*, ed. Terence Ranger and Paul Slack (New York: Cambridge University Press, 1992): 213.

16. Ibid., 236.

17. Ibid., 237.

18. Buzan, Waever, and Wilde, *Security*, 208.

19. Stefan Elbe, "Should HIV/AIDS Be Securitized? The Ethical Dilemmas of Linking HIV/AIDS and Security," *International Studies Quarterly* 50, no. 1 (2006): 120.

20. Ibid., 128.

21. Ibid.

22. "HIV Carriers Face Microchip Implants in Indonesia's Papua Province," *Guardian* (London), November 24, 2008, http://www.theguardian.com/world/2008/nov/24/indonesia-aids.

23. Rita Floyd, "Towards a Consequentialist Evaluation of Security: Bringing Together the Copenhagen and the Welsh Schools of Security Studies," *Review of International Studies* 33, no. 2 (2007): 342.

24. Ibid.

25. See Marc J. Roberts and Michael R. Reich, "Ethical Analysis in Public Health," *The Lancet* 359 (March 23, 2002): 1055–56.

26. Barry Buzan, *People, States, and Fear: An Agenda for International Security Studies in the Post-Cold War Era*, 2nd ed. (London: Harvester Wheatsheaf, 1991), 19.

27. See Sabina Gainotti, Nicola Moran, Carlo Petrini, and Darren Shickle, "Ethical Models Underpinning Responses to Threats to Public Health: A Comparison of Approaches to Communicable Disease Control in Europe," *Bioethics* 22, no. 9 (2008): 466–76.

28. See Margaret P. Battin, Leslie P. Francis, Jay A. Jacobsen, and Charles B. Smith, *The Patient as Victim and Vector: Ethics and Infectious Disease* (Oxford: Oxford University Press, 2009).

29. UN Commission on Human Rights, "Siracusa Principles on the Limitation and Derogation Provisions in the International Covenant on Civil and Political Rights," *Human Rights Quarterly* 7, no. 1 (1985): 6.

30. See Gainotti, Moran, Petrini, and Shickle, "Ethical Models," 470; Ross E.G. Upshur, "Principles for the Justification of Public Health Intervention," *Canadian Journal of Public Health* 93 (2002): 101–3; and Michael J. Selgelid, "A Moderate Pluralist Approach to Public Health Policy and Ethics," *Public Health Ethics* 2, no. 2 (2009): 202.

31. Selgelid, "Ethics and Infectious Disease," 278.

32. Charles B. Smith et al., "Are There Characteristics of Infectious Diseases that Raise Special Ethical Issues?," *Ethics and Infectious Disease*, ed. Michael J. Selgelid, Margaret P. Battin, and Charles B. Smith (Malden, MA: Blackwell, 2006), 21.

33. Ho-fung Hung, "The Politics of SARS: Containing the Perils of Globalization by More Globalization," *Asian Perspective* 28, no. 1 (2004): 41; Erik Eckholm, "SARS Is the Spark for a Riot in China," *New York Times*, April 29, 2003, A1; Jacques deLisle, "SARS, Greater China, and the Pathologies of Globalisation and Transition," *Orbis* 47, no. 4 (2003): 598.

34. Buzan, Waever, and de Wilde, *Security*, 34.

35. This subsection develops ideas that were first raised in a 2013 article: Christian Enemark, "Drug-Resistant Tuberculosis: Security, Ethics and Global Health," *Global Society* 27, no. 2 (2013): 159–77.

36. World Health Organization, *Global Tuberculosis Control: WHO Report 2014*, No. WHO/HTM/TB/2014.08 (2014), chap. 5.

37. World Health Organization, "Tuberculosis," Fact Sheet No. 104, August 2002, http://www.who.int/mediacentre/factsheets/who104/en/print.html.

38. World Health Organization, "Emergence of XDR-TB," September 5, 2006, http://www.who.int/mediacentre/news/notes/2006/np23/en/.

39. World Health Organization, *A Safer Future: Global Public Health Security in the Twenty-First Century*, WHO Report (2007), 53.

40. "TB Poses Security Threat in Russia, Official Says," NewsMedical.net, September 24, 2008, http://www.news-medical.net/news/2008/09/24/41649.aspx.

41. "Ghana Should Declare TB as a National Security Threat—Mr. Gidisu," GhanaWeb.com, March 23, 2010, http://www.ghanaweb.com/GhanaHomePage/health/artikel.php?ID=179057.

42. "South Africa and XDR-TB: Is Forced Isolation the Cure?," IRIN, March 23, 2007, http://pictures.irinnews.org/in-depth/70886/37/south-africa-xdr-tb-is-forced-isolation-the-cure.

43. Adele Baleta, "Forced Isolation of Tuberculosis Patients in South Africa," *The Lancet Infectious Diseases* 7, no. 12 (2007): 771.
44. Zoe Alsop, "Dealing with Drug-Resistant Tuberculosis in Africa," *The Lancet* 372 (September 6, 2008): 793.
45. Fiona Lloyd-Davies, "Life in the Shadow of Deadly New TB," BBC News, November 14, 2008, http://news.bbc.co.uk/2/hi/africa/7729184.stm.
46. Travis C. Porco and Wayne M. Getz, "Controlling Extensively Drug-Resistant Tuberculosis," *The Lancet* 370 (October 27, 2007): 1464.
47. World Health Organization, "Ethical Issues in Tuberculosis Prevention, Care and Control," January 2011, http://www.who.int/tb/publications/ethics_in_tb_fact sheet_28jan11rev.pdf.
48. Chandavarkar, "Plague Panic," 213.
49. World Health Organization, *Guidance on Ethics of Tuberculosis Prevention, Care and Control*, Report No. WHO/HTM/TB/2010.16 (2010), 17.
50. Keertan Dheda and Giovanni B. Migliori, "The Global Rise of Extensively Drug-Resistant Tuberculosis: Is the Time to Bring Back Sanatoria Overdue?," *The Lancet* 379 (February 25, 2012): 773.
51. See Richard Coker, Marianna Thomas, Karen Lock, and Robyn Martin, "Detention and the Evolving Threat of Tuberculosis: Evidence, Ethics, and Law," *Journal of Law, Medicine and Ethics* (Winter 2007): 613.
52. Buzan, Waever, and de Wilde, *Security*, 5.
53. Lawrence O. Gostin and Eric A. Friedman, "A Retrospective and Prospective Analysis of the West African Ebola Virus Disease Epidemic: Robust National Health Systems at the Foundation and an Empowered WHO at the Apex," *The Lancet* 385 (May 9, 2015): 1902.
54. Donald G. McNeil Jr., "Ebola, Killing Scores in Guinea, Threatens Nearby Nations," *New York Times*, March 25, 2014, A3; Andrew Green, "West Africa Struggles to Contain Ebola Outbreak," *The Lancet* 383 (April 5, 2014): 1196.
55. Adam Nossiter, "Ebola Reaches Guinean Capital, Stirring Fears," *New York Times*, April 2, 2014, A4.
56. World Health Organization, "Statement on the First Meeting of the IHR Emergency Committee on the 2014 Ebola Outbreak in West Africa," August 8, 2014, http://www.who.int/mediacentre/news/statements/2014/ebola-20140808/en/.
57. World Health Organization, "No Early End to the Ebola Outbreak," August 14, 2014, http://www.who.int/csr/disease/ebola/overview-20140814/en/.
58. Saliou Samb, Emma Farge, and Angus MacSwan, "Guinean Security Forces Break Up Riot in Ebola-Racked South," Reuters, August 29, 2014, http://www.reuters.com/article/2014/08/29/us-health-ebola-guinea-idUSKBN0GT0ZM 20140829.
59. Centers for Disease Control and Prevention, "CDC Telebriefing on the Update on Ebola Outbreak in West Africa," September 2, 2014, http://www.cdc.gov/media/releases/2014/t0902-ebola-outbreak.html.
60. "Ebola Outbreak 'Threatens Liberia's National Existence,'" BBC News, September 10, 2014, http://www.bbc.co.uk/news/world-africa-29136594.
61. Adam Nossiter, "Lax Quarantine Undercuts Ebola Fight in Africa," *New York Times*, August 5, 2014, A1.

62. Adam Nossiter and Denise Grady, "Africa Presses Effort to Curb Ebola's Spread," *New York Times*, August 1, 2014, A1.

63. Donald G. McNeil Jr., "Using a Tactic Unseen in a Century, Countries Cordon Off Ebola-Racked Areas," *New York Times*, August 13, 2014, A10.

64. Adam Nossiter, "At Heart of Ebola Outbreak, a Village Frozen by Fear and Death," *New York Times*, August 12, 2014, A1; Umaru Fofana and Clair MacDougall, "Sierra Leone, Liberia Deploy Troops as Ebola Toll Hits 887," Reuters, August 5, 2014, http://uk.reuters.com/article/2014/08/04/uk-healh-ebola-africa-idUKKBN0 G41D820140804.

65. Jonathan Paye-Layleh, "Liberia Declares State of Emergency over Ebola Virus," BBC News, August 7, 2014, http://www.bbc.co.uk/news/world-28684561.

66. "Ebola Crisis: Liberia and Sierra Leone Blockades Go Up," BBC News, August 7, 2014, http://www.bbc.co.uk/news/world-africa-28690799.

67. Sarah Latimer, "Police, Residents Clash in Liberian Slum under Ebola Quarantine," *Washington Post*, August 20, 2014, http://www.washingtonpost.com/news/world /wp/2014/08/20/police-residents-clash-in-liberian-slum-under-ebola-quarantine/; Norimitsu Onishi, "As Ebola Grips City, Quarantine Adds to Chaos," *New York Times*, August 29, 2014, A1.

68. Clair MacDougall, "Working, and Playing, to Ease Tensions over an Ebola Quarantine," *New York Times*, May 13, 2015, A7.

69. Gainotti et al., "Ethical Models," 469.

6

BORDER SECURITY AND TRANSNATIONAL CONTAGION

IN MAY 2007 the US government ordered the arrest and isolation of Andrew Speaker, a US citizen who had been diagnosed with XDR-TB infection. The extreme social distancing measure was the first such order issued since 1963, when a smallpox patient in the United States was forcibly isolated. The order was preceded by an attempt by officials to prevent Speaker from traveling across international borders. This kind of biosecurity practice is the focus of the present chapter. Speaker had managed to fly to Europe and then reenter the United States despite his name being placed on the "no fly" list of the Transportation Security Administration (TSA) and official instruction to US Customs and Border Protection officers to detain him.[1] The incident provoked intense political concern about whether the nation's borders, and the personnel and practices that attend them, were sufficiently protective of public health and national security. During hearings before Congress, government officials were accused of failure, Andrew Speaker was accused of having been recklessly indifferent to the health and safety of others, and some lawmakers voiced concern about bioterrorism perpetrated by incoming air passengers. Senator Judd Gregg, for example, warned, "The bigger issue here is . . . what happens if a terrorist who wants to be a martyr, or a group of martyrs, decide to infect themselves and travel?"[2] Representative Christopher Shays described Speaker as "potentially a walking biological weapon . . . no less dangerous because he was determined to be married in Europe than he would have been if he were a terrorist intent on importing . . . bioterrorism."[3] A response was swiftly implemented, and over the following year the TSA's new Do Not Board list (authorized under the Aviation and Transportation Security Act of 2001) prevented the travel of thirty-three other people with suspected or confirmed infectious TB.[4] Henceforth, just as the US government could take the extraordinary measure of restricting freedom of movement for counterterrorism purposes, so too could it now address a public health risk using the same regulatory mechanism. A possible downside of this approach, however, is that the social stigma of having TB might be worsened by associating it so directly with the threat of terrorism. As discussed in the previous chapter, disease-control efforts can be counterproductive if they occasion TB patients to conceal their condition and avoid contact with health authorities. Perhaps, therefore, the government's use of a "no fly" list amounted to negative securitization of TB.

This chapter extends the discussion of the remedy or overkill dilemma beyond the national level and considers the advantages and disadvantages of international bordering as a biosecurity practice. Whether this practice involves monitoring people for infection at entry/exit points or preventing contagion by restricting international travel, there exists an ethical concern to avoid the kind of bordering that is ineffective or counterproductive from a disease-control perspective. To explore this proposition, the relationship between public health, national security, and international borders must be examined. This is a relationship of long standing that might partly explain why some national leaders are quick to invoke the importance of border security when confronting the spread of a dreaded disease. The second section of the chapter focuses on international bordering as it was practiced by some governments during the 2009 H1N1 influenza ("swine flu") pandemic. That experience showed that excessively severe restrictions on cross-border travel can exacerbate rather than mitigate the adverse impact of a contagious disease. In the final section, the remedy or overkill dilemma is further explored in the context of the 2014 Ebola outbreak in West Africa during which some states' negative securitization of the disease took the form of unilateral travel bans. In response, other states acted collectively to "desecuritize" Ebola as a matter of international concern in order to facilitate the provision of medical assistance to people and states in need of it.

PUBLIC HEALTH, NATIONAL SECURITY, AND INTERNATIONAL BORDERING

Borders between nation-states have for a long time been the locus of security practice. For government officials confronting threats and risks of many kinds, there is a strong and understandable temptation to think first about the politically circumscribed territory for which they are responsible. Although the forces of globalization are increasingly challenging the meaning, relevance, and utility of national borders, they can still serve as symbols both for peoples' national identity vis-à-vis the wider world and for governments' outward exercise of national power. Invoking and securing "the border" accords with the often exclusionary logic of security because a sense of *national* security is in large measure experienced in reference to a barrier that putatively divides, distances, or defends the people inside a given territory from the people outside of it. When it comes to infectious diseases, as Elbe has observed, "the widespread perception of microbes as "invaders . . . maps neatly onto a pre-existing idea of national security involving the protection of populations against external threats."[5] Because it is people who carry these microbes, keeping out a dreaded disease can sometimes seem to require keeping out people. Border-based or immigration-related biosecurity measures can thus serve a useful political purpose in assuaging the anxiety of populations inside a given territory. The assurance and expectation, then, is that international borders are meaningful in protecting healthy bodies within from diseased bodies without.

In medieval Europe, priests permanently excluded victims of leprosy ("lepers") not just from local communities but also, as a matter of religion, from the world of the living.[6] This was an ongoing practice in response to a relatively rare disease and, as such, it did not have the same geopolitical significance as did the responses to a great plague that swiftly swept through Europe in the mid-fourteenth century. During this time (1347–50), and in the centuries following the so-called Black Death, the use of sanitary blockades was commonplace. According to Philip Alcabes, "The *cordon sanitaire* contributed to people's sense of identity as a community, town, or nation" by "providing a sense of protection against the ingress of disease."[7] For a period of 160 years, commencing in the early eighteenth century, the Austrian Empire maintained a thousand-mile sanitary cordon "to keep at bay the plague among their Ottoman neighbors."[8] However, it was dread of another bacterial disease (cholera) that occasioned in Europe the most severe attempts to secure national borders—often militarily—against transnational contagion. When cholera moved in waves northwest from South Asia starting in the early nineteenth century, governments rushed to intercept it. For example, an epidemic appeared likely to spread into Moscow in 1830, and "no effort was spared in sequestering the city: a military cordon was drawn, the approaching roads dug up, bridges and ferries destroyed, the city sealed at all but four entrances."[9] The response of neighboring Prussia, according to Peter Baldwin's account, was to establish "an immense military cordon . . . some two hundred miles long and enforced by the efforts of 60,000 troops."[10]

The cholera pandemic that reached Europe in 1865 had spread there from India via the domains of the declining Ottoman Empire, and the arrival of the disease in the Middle East had been facilitated by the Muslim pilgrimage to Mecca. By that time governments in Europe were minded to regard the apparent Ottoman failure to contain disease as a reason to involve themselves in the empire's public health affairs. In the name of "internationalizing public health," as Patrick Zylberman has argued, the powerful states of Europe set about "taking Egypt away from the Sultan in Constantinople."[11] The local authorities in Egypt, under political pressure to allay European fears of cholera, placed in the path of pilgrims "administrative red tape, brutal detentions, obstacles of all kinds."[12] Upon their return to the Red Sea region after visiting Mecca, pilgrims seeking then to reenter Egypt were placed in a beachfront detention station for a period of fifteen to twenty days if a suspected case of cholera was declared on board their vessel. This period was extended following each new case of the disease, which meant pilgrims' confinement could sometimes last up to four months; in these desert conditions they suffered from extreme heat during the day and extreme cold at night. The quarantine station was guarded by soldiers, moreover, and anyone trying to escape it could be shot.[13]

In this particular scenario a person's dangerousness as a (potential) cholera carrier was tied up with his or her dangerousness as a pilgrim, so it is unsurprising that Muslims as a whole came to be unjustly blamed by some Europeans for spreading cholera. Such scapegoating is directly comparable to the way in which fourteenth-century Jews were blamed for the Black Death, and it is partly explicable by reference to any perceived relationship between public health and *national* security. Just as international bordering against cholera generated an expectation that healthy nations would remain free of foreign diseases, so, too, was it prone to fuel people's irrational yet habitual association of foreignness with disease. This racist habit was also evident in 2003 when, due to "a deep-seated stereotype of the Chinese as unhygienic," people of Chinese ethnicity were sometimes blamed for SARS.[14] Likewise, some Mexicans were subjected to discrimination because of swine flu in 2009,[15] and in 2014 some West Africans endured being blamed for Ebola.[16] Scapegoating of this kind clearly compounds the social stigma of disease and potentially increases people's reluctance to engage with authorities' efforts to protect public health. For present purposes, the lesson from history seems to be that if international bordering as a biosecurity practice highlights differences of nationality, it also risks becoming counterproductive to disease control over the long term.

In 1987 it was precisely the US surgeon general's concern to avoid counterproductive measures that reportedly led him to reject a proposal to send all AIDS patients to a former leper colony in Hawaii. There was already at that time a strong stigma against people living with HIV or AIDS. It was not race based but rather attributable to the disease's association with homosexuality and drug use. In the judgment of the surgeon general, the prospect of indefinite isolation—of literally being treated like a leper—would only frighten HIV patients into hiding.[17] A concern about the stigma did not, however, prevent government officials from prohibiting the entry of HIV-positive immigrants into the United States. This prohibition lasted from 1987 until 2009, despite internal criticism that undocumented migrants, fearful of deportation, were being driven "away from public health care, HIV testing and counselling, and treatment programs."[18] The HIV travel ban also attracted international criticism, especially after the IHRs were revised in 2005. The purpose of the regulations, which are legally binding on WHO member states, is

> to prevent, protect against, control and provide a public health response to the international spread of disease in ways that are commensurate with and restricted to public health risks, and which *avoid unnecessary interference with international traffic and trade* (emphasis added).[19]

Inasmuch as the HIV travel ban imposed by the US government was counterproductive to public health, it was difficult to justify it as a *necessary* restriction on international movement.

In the sections that follow, the problem of "unnecessary interference" is discussed in relation to two international-scale outbreaks involving a dreaded disease: the 2009 swine flu pandemic and the 2014 Ebola outbreak in West Africa. In both cases the practice of international bordering was time-critical because they involved a pathogenic microorganism that, unlike the AIDS virus, could spread and kill quickly. As such, these outbreaks were apt to be framed in security terms. The bordering practices that some states implemented against swine flu tended toward the mere monitoring of disease (temperature screening at airports, on-arrival health declarations, etc.). However, the response to the pandemic also included some unilateral restrictions on travel that were implemented against WHO advice that these were unnecessary. This extreme form of international bordering, for which there is ample historical precedent, can often be politically popular but can also give rise to a biosecurity dilemma. On the one hand, travel restrictions intuitively seem a good idea because preventing a person's entry into a country also prevents the entry of any contagious microorganisms inside that person's body. On the other hand, as the 2014 Ebola outbreak in particular showed, an effective response to a disease outbreak might be critically dependent on the free flow of people across international borders.

BORDER SCREENING AND THE SWINE FLU PANDEMIC

For several years prior to the 2009 swine flu pandemic, governments around the world had been concerned about and preparing for the possibility of acute, large-scale outbreaks of deadly infectious diseases. The emergence and spread of SARS

in 2003 was a dramatic reminder of the difficulty of controlling a disease without drugs and vaccines. The human toll from SARS was ultimately only 8,098
reported cases with 774 deaths, but the newness of the disease was grounds for
initial fears that the toll might be far worse.[20] The outbreak of a disease hitherto
unknown to medical science was significant also because it necessitated, for the
first time in many decades, the widespread use of nonpharmaceutical disease-
control measures both domestically and internationally.[21] Moreover, SARS
foreshadowed another, somewhat greater microbial risk against which pharmaceuticals would not be immediately available: the emergence of a new subtype
of human-to-human transmissible influenza virus. Such a virus (H1N1 "swine
flu") emerged in 2009, but in the meantime political and scientific attention
had been focused on the pandemic risk posed by another: the H5N1 "bird flu"
virus. After the appearance in early 2004 of a mysterious disease killing chickens
in Vietnam, H5N1 swept through poultry flocks across East Asia. The following
year it spread westward and caused outbreaks in India, the Middle East, Europe,
and Africa. As a problem of animal health, H5N1 was bad enough, but its significance for public health lay in its potential to mutate into a pandemic form.
The H5N1 virus has repeatedly managed to jump species and successfully infect
humans, and every instance of this is a mutation opportunity. At the time of
writing there had been 844 confirmed human cases of H5N1 influenza across
sixteen countries since 2003, including 449 deaths (a global average case-fatality
rate of around 53 percent).[22]

In anticipation of an imminent influenza pandemic, in 2005 the WHO
drafted its Global Influenza Preparedness Plan. This document was informed
by the recent experience of SARS and advised against using some of the border-
based biosecurity measures that some governments had implemented in 2003.
In particular the WHO advised states against screening incoming travelers at
points of entry: "Due to lack of proven health benefit, [this] practice should be
permitted (for political reasons, to promote public confidence) but not encouraged."[23] It was a message later reinforced by the ethical advice that "plans related
to travel restrictions and border controls should . . . respect, to the extent possible, the individual right to freedom of movement."[24] From a biosecurity perspective, the lesson of the SARS outbreak had shown that infrared thermal image
scanners (to detect body temperatures above 38 degrees Celsius) yielded negligi-
ble public health benefits but were costly and inconvenient. Although thirty-five
million people had been screened for SARS at airports in four Asian countries,
not one case of the disease was detected.[25] In Canada, where around C$7.5
million was spent on airport screening measures and eight hundred thousand
people were thermally scanned, five SARS-infected people still managed to enter

the country because they were not showing symptoms of disease at the time of entry.[26] Despite this experience, and contrary to the WHO's scientific advice, in November 2005 Shanghai's Pudong International Airport began using thermal scanners to screen international passengers for symptoms of influenza.[27] China had suffered more than any other country from the health and economic effects of SARS, so perhaps this screening was being done "for political reasons, to promote public confidence."[28] If so, and because the WHO's position was that "[this] practice should be permitted,"[29] the action probably did not amount to "unnecessary interference with international traffic."[30] However, when a pandemic influenza virus later emerged and started spreading around the world, the Chinese government's international bordering practices were, like those of some other governments, sometimes much more severe. Specifically, the international travel bans that were unilaterally imposed in response to swine flu in 2009 were emergency measures beyond rules that would otherwise bind (the IHRs). To the extent that these bans were counterproductive to disease control, they exemplified negative securitization of pandemic influenza.

The worst influenza pandemic of the twentieth century, the Spanish flu of 1918–19, killed around 50 million people worldwide. Subsequent pandemics in 1957 and 1968 were much less deadly, causing 2 million and 1 million deaths, respectively. The widespread concern about the mutation of H5N1 bird flu tended to focus on the prospect of a severe, "1918-style" pandemic. The WHO seemed to adopt this expectation as well, and in 2007 its annual World Health Report described pandemic influenza as "the most feared security threat."[31] As discussed earlier, the political framing of pandemic influenza in security terms sometimes garnered attention, effort, and resources for implementing a swift and robust response. In hindsight, however, a security-oriented posture of preparedness might have increased the likelihood that governments would overreact to an influenza pandemic, which in the end turned out to be mild. The 2009 swine flu was just such a pandemic, and some governments exhibited a determination to use border-based disease-control mechanisms despite WHO advice that these were ineffective and unjustifiably disruptive.

On April 6, 2009, health officials in the Mexican state of Veracruz raised an alert over a respiratory disease outbreak in the town of La Gloria (250 kilometers east of Mexico City). Later that month, in the United States the CDC determined that two children in adjacent counties in southern California had illnesses (dating from late March) caused by infection with a new subtype of H1N1 influenza virus. On April 23, after a conference call with US health officials, Mexican health minister José Angel Córdova telephoned President Felipe Calderón, reportedly saying, "Mr. President, I need to see you urgently. It's a matter of national security."[32] Human-to-human transmission of a new subtype of influenza virus had been confirmed. Two days later the WHO declared the outbreak, which became known as "swine flu," to be a PHEIC, and on April 27 it raised the pandemic alert level from phase 3 to phase 4 (on a 6-phased approach to preparedness and response) because *sustained* human-to-human transmission of the new virus had by then been confirmed.[33] At the same time, though, the organization recommended the abandonment of efforts to contain the spread of disease. WHO deputy director-general Keiji Fukuda explained, "Because the virus is already quite widespread in different locations, containment is not a feasible option."[34] On April 29 the WHO raised its alert level from phase 4 to phase 5 (because human-to-human transmission in two or more countries had been confirmed), but by then US health officials had taken the lead in assuming that a pandemic was fully under way. On the same day as the WHO made its phase 5 announcement, Homeland Security secretary Janet Napolitano declared that the US government was taking action, "as if this were stage [phase] 6," because it was trying to "stay ahead of whatever number WHO assigns."[35] Her explanation was emblematic of the attitude of several governments at the time, that national disease-control efforts should not be constrained by WHO guidance.

The guidance issued by WHO spokesman Gregory Hartl at the end of April 2009 was unequivocal: "Border controls do not work. Screening doesn't work. If a person has been exposed or infected . . . the person might not be symptomatic at the airport. . . . SARS was a huge learning experience."[36] Yet his advice was spectacularly ignored as government after government rushed to engage in international bordering in a vain attempt to contain a virus that, according to the WHO, could no longer be contained. Within the space of a week Argentina, Canada, Cuba, Ecuador, and Peru banned flights from Mexico. The US embassy in Mexico City suspended visa-processing services, Japan stopped issuing visas to Mexicans who arrived in the country, and Singapore used public health orders to quarantine (for one week) anyone arriving from Mexico.[37] Entry by sea was sometimes prohibited, too, and the government of Haiti turned away a Mexican aid ship carrying 77 tons of rice, fertilizer, and emergency food kits even though, according to Mexican officials, screening of the ship's crew revealed no signs of influenza.[38] Later the same month health authorities in Australia instituted a rule reminiscent of the forty-day waiting period (*quarantina*) imposed on all ships arriving at the port of Venice at the time of the Black Death. The chief health officer of New South Wales announced: "We will be treating all cruise ships as if they had swine flu on board and taking appropriate responses . . . [including] not letting people off the ship until we have absolutely cleared swine flu being on it."[39]

The international bordering practiced by the government of China was the most severe of all, and a senior Chinese health official suggested in late 2009 that a national security imperative had driven his government's actions: "If these strict measures had not been taken, and if there had been a sudden outbreak of the disease, there would have been a huge panic among the Chinese population."[40] Nevertheless, some of China's border-based biosecurity practices departed the furthest from WHO advice (and from the IHRs), and the counterproductive effect of this suggests that negative securitization was taking place. Perhaps of greatest significance was the decision in early May 2009 to quarantine seventy Mexican nationals who had entered China on the same flight as a man who was diagnosed with swine flu.[41] Mexican foreign minister Patricia Espinosa complained publicly that "Mexican citizens showing no signs at all of being ill [had] been isolated under unacceptable conditions," and she described the quarantine imposed by the Chinese officials as "discriminatory" and "without foundation."[42] The diplomatic row reached its height on May 5, 2009, when the Mexican government sent a chartered airplane to retrieve Mexicans who had been quarantined in Shanghai, Beijing, Guangzhou, and Hong Kong.[43] The previous day, in an address to the nation, President Calderón probably had China in mind when he said:

> We are defending not only Mexicans but all the human beings in the world that could catch this new disease. And we will be able to fight this battle more easily if the world collaborates with us. . . . on behalf of Mexicans, I would ask all countries that have done so, to stop taking actions that only damage Mexico and fail to stop the spread of the disease.[44]

WHO director-general Margaret Chan supported this request, issuing a "strong plea" for countries to "refrain from introducing measures that are economically and socially disruptive, yet have no scientific justification and bring no clear public health benefit."[45] Eventually the evident ineffectiveness and counterproductive effect of international bordering occasioned governments to shift their focus toward diagnosing and treating swine flu cases. However, the experience of responding to this influenza pandemic appeared not to diminish the willingness of some governments to regard well-policed national borders as meaningful barriers to transnational contagion. Five years later the problem of negative securitization *qua* "unnecessary interference with international traffic" arose again in the context of an Ebola outbreak in West Africa. When disease-control efforts there were thus critically undermined, part of the political remedy was to remove Ebola from the realm of *national* security policy and so facilitate the cross-border movement of people who were willing and able to help.

TRAVEL RESTRICTIONS AND EBOLA IN WEST AFRICA

In late June 2014, by which time the Ebola outbreak then ongoing in West Africa had become the largest ever in terms of the number of reported cases and deaths, WHO Africa Region director Luis Sambo declared:

> This is no longer a country-specific outbreak, but a sub-regional crisis that requires firm action. WHO is gravely concerned of the on-going cross-border transmission into neighbouring countries as well as the potential for further international spread. There is an urgent need to intensify response efforts . . . this is the only way that the outbreak will be effectively addressed.[46]

The Ebola virus does not transmit easily (e.g., through the air) so it is relatively easy to contain using basic infection-control measures. Moreover, supportive medical care (such as rehydrating those with diarrhea or vomiting) can improve one's chances of surviving the disease. In the absence of a vaccine or therapeutic drug, therefore, the best approach to Ebola relief in West Africa was to insert a large number of capable, adequately supplied medical personnel into the situation to treat illness and prevent infection. To that end, in late July 2014 Margaret Chan announced a $100 million plan to send more experts and supplies to the region.[47] Such an approach was stymied, however, by unilateral decisions by some governments to restrict or prohibit travel to and from the worst-affected countries (Guinea, Liberia, and Sierra Leone).

On August 8, 2014, when the WHO declared the Ebola outbreak to be a PHEIC and advised states with active Ebola transmission to declare a national emergency, its advice to *all* states was "There should be no general ban on international travel."[48] The president of Nigeria responded by declaring a national emergency in his country, where only two people had died of Ebola.[49] One of those victims, though, had been a man who traveled by airplane from Liberia to the Nigerian capital, Lagos, and popular fear had erupted at the notion that Ebola might spread through the heavily populated city.[50] The Nigerian government had already acted in a way that soon set a trend for establishing international *cordons sanitaires* against Ebola. In late July 2014 Nigerian airline Arik Air suspended all flights to Liberia and Sierra Leone;[51] Nigeria's health minister afterward warned that "everyone in the world is at risk" because of air travel.[52] The following month, several other West African countries, including Ivory Coast and Senegal, banned all travel to and from Guinea, Liberia, and Sierra Leone.[53] The Kenyan government announced that Kenya was also closing its borders to travelers from those three countries,[54] describing its decision as "in line with the recognition of the extraordinary measures urgently required to contain the Ebola outbreak in West Africa."[55] Air France suspended flights to Freetown, Sierra Leone, on the recommendation of the French government,[56] and the South African government announced that noncitizens arriving from Ebola-affected areas of West Africa would not be allowed into South Africa.[57]

The logic of travel bans seemed to be that if *some* people traveling from West Africa *might* be carrying the Ebola virus, the prevention of inward travel by *all* such people would reduce the Ebola importation risk to zero. However, there is no scientific basis for adopting this extremely risk-averse approach, which is why the WHO repeatedly advised against travel bans.[58] Such bans, when they were implemented anyway, therefore appeared to contravene the IHR rule against *unnecessary* interference with international traffic. Or, to use the terms of securitization theory, the travel bans imposed in an attempt to achieve zero risk of Ebola transmission were "emergency measures beyond rules that would otherwise bind."[59]

Because these bans promised to be counterproductive to public health (in West Africa, at least), they arguably constituted negative securitization. The placing of restrictions on the insertion of medical personnel and supplies into Ebola-affected countries increased the risk that local people would try to leave those countries in search of safety or treatment. In turn, this increased the risk of the disease spreading to other countries ill-equipped to cope with Ebola.[60] As the Liberian foreign minister observed at the time, "There is a panicked reaction across the globe, but disproportionate actions [travel bans] will only compound the problem here and limit our ability to contain the virus."[61] Apparently the faltering response to Ebola needed to be released from the stranglehold of "panic politics," and the forum for arranging this happened to be the UN Security Council. In the month of September 2014 it was the turn of the United States to hold the presidency of the council, and the United States used its position to propose a resolution aimed at unplugging the flow of medical assistance to Ebola-stricken West Africa.

By the end of August 2014, and despite their evident appetite for *cordons sanitaires* within their own territories (see chapter 5), the presidents of Guinea, Liberia, and Sierra Leone were pleading for international travel bans to be lifted. At an Economic Community of West African States meeting in Ghana they were supported by Ghanaian president John Mahama, who warned that "excessive restrictions of travel and border closures will adversely affect the economies of the sub-region."[62] On September 8 the African Union issued a statement on the Ebola outbreak that urged member states "to respect the principle of free movement, and to ensure that all restrictions are in line with recommendations from the relevant international organisations."[63] A week later the UN secretary-general transmitted to the Security Council a letter he had received from the presidents of Guinea, Liberia, and Sierra Leone (dated August 29, 2014). The presidents complained therein about "virtual economic sanctions and trade embargoes that will end up aggravating the effect of the outbreak on our economies and stifling attempts to control the [Ebola] epidemic." The "blanket travel bans" implemented by some other states would, they argued, make it "impossible to bring in the international expertise and supplies required to end the outbreak." The presidents therefore urgently requested, in the form of a "resolution," the "intervention of the United Nations with our neighbours far and near to end the sanctions."[64]

When the Security Council convened on September 18, its president (the US representative) described the problem to be addressed:

> Precisely at the moment when a robust, united intervention was needed, some countries started to seal their borders. This reaction, driven by a mix of fear and the desire to protect one's own citizens from the virus's spread, was understandable. The problem is that while isolation is effective and indeed necessary for dealing with individuals who may have been exposed to Ebola, it is utterly counterproductive when applied to entire countries. It deprives them of the very resources they need to bring the virus under control.[65]

Some lingering panic was at that time still evident in the Nigerian representative's subsequent hyperbolic description of Ebola as an "apocalyptic virus" that posed a threat "to the entire globe."[66] However, as the debate in the council proceeded, other representatives emphasized the need for some panic-stricken governments to abandon their counterproductive response practices. Guinea's foreign minister argued that "border closures, flight restrictions, stigmatization of victims, isolation of affected countries and repatriation of their citizens constitute a weapon that is more dangerous than the scourge being combatted."[67] The foreign minister of Sierra Leone said, "To those countries that, through panicked reactions, have closed their borders and cancelled flights and shipping arrangements, I want to join my colleagues from Liberia and Guinea to plead for a return to normalcy."[68] His was a plea, in other words, to remove the issue of Ebola from the "agenda of panic politics" so that it may be "better handled within normal politics."[69] The UK representative agreed, stating,

> It is important to remember that Ebola is a preventable and containable disease, but only if we all work together to stop it and confront the fear and stigma associated with the disease. We must not let fear dictate the response; instead, we must act.[70]

The catalyst for such action was Resolution 2177, in which the Security Council expressed concern about "the detrimental effect of the isolation of the affected countries as a result of trade and travel restrictions imposed on and to the affected countries."[71] Accordingly, the council called on UN member states "to lift general travel and border restrictions" and "to facilitate the delivery of assistance, including qualified, specialized and trained personnel and supplies, in response to the Ebola outbreak to the affected countries."[72] The Security Council thereby denounced the emergency measure of travel bans as unnecessary (and, by implication, a violation of the IHRs) and encouraged an increased international provision of medical resources that would, in turn, reduce the pressure felt by governments in West Africa to resort to mass quarantine. As against some states' national-level, harmful border-based responses to the Ebola outbreak, Resolution 2177 could perhaps be regarded as a positive, international-level desecuritizing move. Effectively, and for the sake of public health, the Security Council had situated the response to Ebola *outside* the realm of national security policy.

The practical effect of this move was not, however, to completely remove every impediment to the free flow of medical personnel willing to assist disease victims in West Africa. In the United States itself, and despite the federal government's international leadership on urging the repeal of travels bans, there was continuing domestic political pressure to close all US borders against the dreaded Ebola. The pressure increased within days of the passage of Resolution 2177, when the contagion risk associated with travel to and from Ebola-affected areas was for the first time realized outside Africa. In late September 2014 a Spanish nurse in Madrid became the first person known to have contracted the Ebola virus in a non-African country. She had helped care for an Ebola patient who had been transported from Sierra Leone to Spain on September 22, and she had also helped with the burial of the patient's body after he died.[73] Soon afterward, the first case of Ebola in the United States occurred in a man who had earlier traveled from Liberia to Texas. In response, CDC director Thomas Frieden offered the assurance "I have no doubt that we will control this importation, or this case of Ebola, so that it does not spread widely in this country."[74] However, Louisiana governor Bobby Jindal responded by advocating the grounding of airplanes "to protect our people,"[75] while US Senate candidate Terri Lynn Land called for "a travel ban . . . to make sure we do not (have) any more cases come into the United States."[76] President Barack Obama resisted these and many other calls for a travel ban, but in early October 2014 the CDC did establish additional layers of on-arrival medical screening at the five US airports that receive over 94 percent of travelers from Guinea, Liberia, and Sierra Leone.[77]

International bordering in the form of entry screening is of dubious value from a public health perspective. Nevertheless, in the context of the 2014 Ebola outbreak, it probably did not constitute unnecessary interference with international traffic. By contrast, the counterproductive effect of a border-based measure that followed—mandatory quarantine of returning US health workers—is more readily characterized as negative securitization of Ebola. Soon after the CDC moved to intensify airport screening, one US doctor who had returned from Guinea was diagnosed with the disease in New York.[78] After it emerged that he had moved around the city in the days before he tested positive for Ebola, the governors of New York and neighboring New Jersey quickly introduced mandatory twenty-one-day quarantine for returned travelers (including health workers) who had had direct contact with Ebola patients in West Africa. The governors reportedly did this because they judged the CDC's requirement—quarantine for *symptomatic* travelers only—as inadequate.[79] Illinois governor Pat Quinn followed suit, describing quarantine as "too important to be voluntary."[80] Similar measures were soon enacted in Connecticut, Georgia, California, Maine, Louisiana, and Florida.[81] In response to the governors' actions, the US ambassador to the United Nations, Samantha Power, told NBC News:

> The American people as a whole and the US government, all of us need to make clear what these health workers mean to us and how much we value their service. We need to find a way when they come home that they are treated like conquering heroes and not stigmatized for the tremendous work that they've done.[82]

As a biosecurity practice, mandatory quarantine in this instance lacked a scientific basis, it implied (erroneously) that asymptomatic people returning from West Africa posed a danger to others, and it was effectively a disincentive for health workers to volunteer to join the fight against Ebola in West Africa. Nevertheless, it was a measure aimed at reducing the risk of disease transmission, and a valid question is, What might have happened had the returning doctor become symptomatic and *not* checked in to a hospital? With the US public deeply concerned about Ebola transmission at the time, the political leaders who implemented mandatory quarantine appeared to have made a judgment call.[83] When faced with a biosecurity dilemma, they judged that the benefit of conspicuously doing more to try to stop the disease from spreading (that is, the remedy) outweighed the harm associated with a heavy-handed approach (the overkill).

CONCLUSION

In a 2007 article about pandemic influenza, Kelley Lee and David Fidler warned that "public officials may feel compelled to adopt measures to demonstrate to domestic constituencies that they are 'doing something.'"[84] This might explain why, on April 30, 2009, Australia's health minister announced that thermal scanners would start screening inward travelers for swine flu, saying, "It's all about us taking additional precautions to try to delay the entry of this disease into Australia."[85] The scientific advice of the WHO was to not bother with bordering practices of this kind. Yet the political temptation to act was strong, and doing too much was perhaps less blameworthy than doing too little. Two years previously, when CDC director Julie Gerberding had announced the compulsory isolation of Andrew Speaker on suspicion of XDR-TB infection, her explanation was, "We felt it was our responsibility to err on the side of abundant caution."[86] The phrase "abundant caution" later featured frequently in official utterances regarding Ebola in the United States, and yet there appeared to be little public concern about the downsides of exercising more caution than is necessary.[87] The potential problem when a remedy or overkill dilemma arises is that a well-intentioned but ineffective biosecurity practice will do more harm than good. When a biosecurity practice is border-based and thus has international implications, it is arguably even more important to avoid the ethical problem of unjustly restricting people's freedom of movement.

Historically there is a political relationship between public health, national security, and international bordering, and to this day the maintenance of that relationship is politically appealing to some government leaders. This might explain why, even despite scientific advice to the contrary, these leaders continue to regard "border security" as meaningful when confronting the spread of a dreaded disease. Pandemic influenza is one such dreaded disease. However, the 2009 swine flu experience showed that severe restrictions on cross-border travel served to hinder national and international public health responses. As individual governments flailed wildly to protect their populations against an uncontainable contagion, swine flu became engulfed in the panic politics of security. Panic occurred again during the 2014 Ebola outbreak in West Africa, when some states' negative securitization of the disease took the form of unilateral travel bans. Fortunately, the US government acted to quell the tendency to adopt a siege mentality, and the passage of Security Council Resolution 2177 relieved the political pressure for implementing desperate, unnecessary, and counterproductive measures. Individual states, whose travel bans contravened the IHR rule against unnecessary interference with international traffic, had been engaged in negative securitization at the national level. Thus the passage of Resolution 2177 could be regarded as a positive, international-level desecuritizing move.

In taking an excessively self-interested, beggar-thy-neighbor approach to disease-control, some states perpetuate the false and harmful message that a deadly and contagious disease is not a globally shared problem. From a public health perspective, appealing to national security might be a good way of focusing national attention and resources. However, given the increasing interdependence of states and the collective vulnerability of their populations to infectious diseases, the better approach to transnational contagion might be cooperation rather than competition. Accordingly, the focus of the next chapter shifts from national border security to "global health security." The problem of how to justly prioritize efforts and allocate resources against a dreaded disease can be an immediate one when a particular disease outbreak is happening (remedy or overkill), but it can also manifest over the long term in institutionalized health governance arrangements at the international and national level. This is the fourth kind of biosecurity dilemma: "attention or neglect."

NOTES

1. Wendy Parmet, "Legal Power and Legal Rights—Isolation and Quarantine in the Case of Drug-Resistant Tuberculosis," *New England Journal of Medicine* 375, no. 5 (2007): 433; Kathleen Swendiman and Nancy Lee Jones, "Extensively Drug-Resistant Tuberculosis (XDR-TB): Quarantine and Isolation," US Department of State, Congressional Research Service Report No. RS22672 (June 5, 2007), http://fpc.state.gov/documents/organization/86251.pdf.
2. "Gregg Wants More Answers on TB Security Breach," *Boston Globe*, June 12, 2007, available to subscribers to the Factiva database http://global.factiva.com/aa/?ref=APRS000020070612e36c00du1&pp=1&fcpil=en&napc=S&sa_from (accessed July 20, 2016).
3. Johanna Neuman and Joel Havemann, "Lawmaker Says US 'Dodged a Bullet' in TB Case," *Los Angeles Times*, June 6, 2007, http://www.latimes.com/travel/la-trw-na-tb7jun07-story.html.
4. Amanda Gardner, "U.S. Barred 33 TB-Infected People from Flying over Past Year," ABC News, September 19, 2008, http://abcnews.go.com/Health/Healthday/story?id=5836417; "Federal Air Travel Restrictions for Public Health Purposes—United States, June 2007–May 2008," *Morbidity and Mortality Weekly Report*, September 19, 2008, http://www.cdc.gov/mmwr/preview/mmwrhtml/mm5737a1.htm.
5. Stefan Elbe, "Should Health Professionals Play the Global Health Security Card?," *The Lancet* 378 (July 16, 2011): 220.
6. Matthew Daly, "Medical Necessity as a Defense for Crimes against Humanity: An Examination of the Molokai Transfers," *Arizona Journal of International and Comparative Law* 24, no. 3 (2007): 656.
7. Philip Alcabes, *Dread: How Fear and Fantasy Have Fueled Epidemics from the Black Death to Avian Flu* (New York: Public Affairs, 2009), 43.
8. Peter Baldwin, *Contagion and the State in Europe, 1830–1930* (Cambridge: Cambridge University Press, 2005), 41.
9. Ibid., 43.
10. Ibid.
11. Patrick Zylberman, "Civilizing the State: Borders, Weak States, and International Health in Modern Europe," in *Medicine at the Border: Disease, Globalization and*

Security, 1850 to the Present, ed. Alison Bashford (Hampshire, UK: Palgrave Macmillan, 2006), 33–34.

12. Ibid., 25.

13. Ibid., 25–26.

14. Ho-fung Hung, "The Politics of SARS: Containing the Perils of Globalization by More Globalization," *Asian Perspective* 28, no. 1 (2004): 33.

15. Marc Lacey and Andrew Jacobs, "Even as Fears of Flu Ebb, Mexicans Feel Stigma," *New York Times*, May 5, 2009, A1.

16. Rebecca Davis, "'I Am a Liberian, Not a Virus': West Africans Hit Back against Ebola Stigma," *Guardian* (London), October 22, 2014, http://www.theguardian.com/world/2014/oct/22/ebola-liberia-not-virus-stigma.

17. Daly, "Medical Necessity," 656.

18. Amy L. Fairchild and Eileen A. Tynan, "Policies of Containment: Immigration in the Era of AIDS," *American Journal of Public Health* 84, no. 12 (1994): 2018.

19. World Health Organization, *International Health Regulations (2005)*, 2nd ed. (Geneva: World Health Organization, 2008), article 2.

20. World Health Organization, "Summary of Probable SARS Cases with Onset of Illness from 1 November 2002 to 31 July 2003," September 26, 2003, http://www.who.int/csr/sars/country/table2003_09_23/en/.

21. See Christian Enemark, *Disease and Security: Natural Plagues and Biological Weapons in East Asia* (Abingdon, UK: Routledge, 2007), 27–40.

22. World Health Organization, "Cumulative Number of Confirmed Human Cases of Avian Influenza A(H5N1) Reported to WHO," October 15, 2015, http://www.who.int/influenza/human_animal_interface/H5N1_cumulative_table_archives/en/.

23. World Health Organization, *WHO Global Influenza Preparedness Plan: The Role of WHO and Recommendations for National Measures before and during Pandemics*, Report No. WHO/CDS/CSR/GIP/2005.5 (2005), 45. See also World Health Organization Writing Group, "Nonpharmaceutical Interventions for Pandemic Influenza, International Measures," *Emerging Infectious Diseases* 12, no. 1 (2006): 86.

24. World Health Organization, *Ethical Considerations in Developing a Public Health Response to Pandemic Influenza*, Report. No. WHO/CDS/EPR/GIP/2007.2 (2007), 10.

25. "Comments from the Center for Biosecurity of UPMC on the National Strategy for Pandemic Influenza: Implementation Plan," *Biosecurity and Bioterrorism* 4, no. 3 (2006): 322.

26. Ronald K. St John et al., "Border Screening for SARS," *Emerging Infectious Diseases* 11, no. 1 (2005): 9; Claire Hooker, "Drawing the Lines: Danger and Risk in the Age of SARS," in *Medicine at the Border: Disease, Globalization and Security, 1850 to the Present*, ed. Alison Bashford (Hampshire, UK: Palgrave Macmillan, 2006), 186.

27. "Arrivals Screened for Bird Flu," *Sydney Morning Herald*, November 29, 2005, http://www.smh.com.au/articles/2005/11/29/1133026444587.html.

28. World Health Organization, *WHO Global Influenza Preparedness Plan*, 45.

29. Ibid.

30. World Health Organization, *International Health Regulations*.

31. *A Safer Future: Global Public Health Security in the Twenty-First Century*, World Health Report 2007 (Geneva: World Health Organization, 2007), 45.

32. "How Scientists Swung into Full Virus Alert," *Weekend Australian* (Sydney), May 2–3, 2009, 14.

33. See World Health Organization, *WHO Global Influenza Preparedness Plan*, 2.

34. Donald G. McNeil Jr., "W.H.O. Issues Higher Alert on Swine Flu, with Advice," *New York Times*, April 28, 2009, A10.

35. Dan Childs, Ammu Kannampilly and Stephen Splane, "Pandemic 'Imminent': WHO Raises Swine Flu Pandemic Alert Level to 5," ABC News, April 29, 2009, http://abcnews.go.com/Health/SwineFlu/story?id=7456439&page=1.

36. "We Can't Halt Spread, WHO Admits, as More Nations Hit," *Australian* (Sydney), April 29, 2009, 9.

37. Lacey and Jacobs, "Even as Fears of Flu Ebb," A1; Rob Stein, "Experts Study Differences in Flu's Severity," *Washington Post*, April 29, 2009, http://www.washingtonpost.com/wp-dyn/content/article/2009/04/28/AR2009042800757.html; "First Countries Suspend Flights to and from Mexico," *Age* (Melbourne), April 29, 2009, http://www.theage.com.au/world/first-countries-suspend-flights-to-and-from-mexico-20090428-am8g; Bryan Walsh, "Why Border Controls Can't Keep Out the Flu Virus," *Time*, April 30, 2009, http://content.time.com/time/health/article/0,8599,1894786,00.html; "Mexico to Shut Down for Five Days," *Weekend Australian* (Sydney), May 2–3, 2009, 15.

38. Thomas H. Maugh II, "Mexico City Reemerges from H1N1 Threat," *Los Angeles Times*, May 7, 2009, http://articles.latimes.com/2009/may/07/science/sci-swine-flu7.

39. "All Cruise Ships in NSW to Be Treated as Having Swine Flu Onboard," *Sydney Morning Herald*, May 28, 2009, http://www.smh.com.au/national/all-cruise-ships-in-nsw-to-be-treated-as-having-swine-flu-onboard-20090528-bnce.

40. Edward Wong, "China's Tough Flu Measures Appear to Be Effective," *New York Times*, November 12, 2009, A3.

41. "Five New UK Flu Cases Confirmed," BBC News, May 5, 2009, http://news.bbc.co.uk/1/hi/world/americas/8033089.stm.

42. Rory Carroll and Tania Branigan, "Mexico Complains of Swine Flu Backlash," *Guardian* (London), May 3, 2009, http://www.theguardian.com/world/2009/may/03/mexico-swine-flu-backlash.

43. Tania Branigan, Julian Border, and Jo Tuckman, "Swine Flu: Mexican Citizens Flown Back from China after Being Held in Hotels," *Guardian* (London), May 5, 2009, http://www.theguardian.com/world/2009/may/05/swine-flu-china-mexico.

44. William Branigin and Ceci Connolly, "Officials Confirm Second U.S. Swine Flu Death," *Washington Post*, May 5, 2009, http://www.washingtonpost.com/wp-dyn/content/article/2009/05/05/AR2009050501905.html.

45. Margaret Chan, "H1N1 Influenza Situation," World Health Organization, May 4, 2009, http://www.who.int/dg/speeches/2009/influenza_a_h1n1_situation_20090504/en/.

46. James Gallagher, "'Drastic Action' Needed on Ebola," BBC News, June 26, 2014, http://www.bbc.co.uk/news/health-28033027.

47. "Ebola Crisis: Virus Spreading Too Fast, Says WHO," BBC News, August 1, 2014, http://www.bbc.co.uk/news/world-africa-28610112; Adam Nossiter and Denise Grady, "Africa Presses Effort to Curb Ebola's Spread," *New York Times*, August 1, 2014, A1.

48. World Health Organization, "Statement on the First Meeting of the IHR Emergency Committee on the 2014 Ebola Outbreak in West Africa," August 8, 2014, http://www.who.int/mediacentre/news/statements/2014/ebola-20140808/en/.

49. "Ebola Outbreak: Nigeria Declares National Emergency," BBC News, August 9, 2014, http://www.bbc.co.uk/news/world-africa-28715939.

50. Tom Cocks, "Ebola Outbreak: Fears for Lagos—A Vast City of 21 Million 'Perfect for the Virus to Spread,'" *Independent* (London), August 13, 2014, http://www.independent.co.uk/news/world/africa/ebola-outbreak-fears-for-lagos--a-vast-city-of-21-million-perfect-for-the-virus-to-spread-9667377.html.

51. "Ebola Outbreak: Liberia Shuts Most Border Points," BBC News, July 28, 2014, http://www.bbc.co.uk/news/world-africa-28522824.

52. Johnathan Paye-Layleh, "Liberia Declares State of Emergency over Ebola Virus," BBC News, August 7, 2014, http://www.bbc.co.uk/news/world-28684561.

53. "Ebola Outbreak: West Africans Back Lifting Travel Bans," BBC News, August 29, 2014, http://www.bbc.co.uk/news/world-africa-28977134.

54. "Kenya Bars Travellers from Ebola-Hit Nations," Al Jazeera, August 16, 2014, http://www.aljazeera.com/news/africa/2014/08/kenya-bars-travellers-from-ebola-hit-nations-2014816211523680238.html.

55. Johnathan Paye-Layleh, "Ebola Fears Heightened in Liberia as Clinic Looted," *USA Today*, August 17, 2014, http://www.usatoday.com/story/news/world/2014/08/17/west-africa-liberia-ebola/14195347/.

56. Robert Wall, "Air France Suspends Flights to Freetown, Sierra Leone over Ebola Outbreak," *Wall Street Journal*, August 27, 2014, http://www.wsj.com/articles/air-france-suspends-flights-to-freetown-sierra-leone-over-ebola-outbreak-1409150478.

57. "Ebola Travel: South Africa Bans Incomers from West Africa," BBC News, August 21, 2014, http://www.bbc.co.uk/news/world-africa-28879020.

58. World Health Organization, "Statement on Travel and Transport in Relation to Ebola Virus Disease Outbreak," August 18, 2014, http://www.who.int/mediacentre/news/statements/2014/ebola-travel-trasport/en/.

59. Barry Buzan, Ole Waever, and Jaap de Wilde, *Security: A New Framework for Analysis* (Boulder, CO: Lynne Rienner, 1998), 5.

60. Jennifer B. Nuzzo, Anita J. Cicero, Richard Waldhorn, and Thomas V. Inglesby, "Travel Bans Will Increase the Damage Wrought by Ebola," *Biosecurity and Bioterrorism* 12, no. 6 (2014): 307.

61. Caelainn Hogan, "WHO Cautions against Ebola-Related Travel Restrictions," *Washington Post*, August 19, 2014, http://www.washingtonpost.com/national/health-science/2014/08/19/83da2974-26f2-11e4-8593-da634b334390_story.html.

62. "Ebola Outbreak: West Africans Back Lifting Travel Bans," BBC News, August 29, 2014, http://www.bbc.co.uk/news/world-africa-28977134.

63. Media release quoted in Patrick M. Eba, "Ebola and Human Rights in West Africa," *The Lancet* 384 (December 13, 2014): 2092.

64. United Nations, Security Council Resolution S/2014/669, September 15, 2014.

65. United Nations, Security Council Resolution S/PV.7268, September 18, 2014, 8.

66. Ibid., 9.

67. Ibid., 24.

68. Ibid., 27.

69. See Buzan, Waever, and de Wilde, *Security*, 34.

70. United Nations, Security Council Resolution S/PV.7268, September 18, 2014, 17.
71. United Nations, Security Council Resolution S/RES/2177, September 18, 2014, 2, 4.
72. Ibid., 4.
73. J. Manuel Parra, Octavio J. Salmerón, and María Velasco, "The First Case of Ebola Virus Disease Acquired outside Africa," *New England Journal of Medicine* 371, no. 25 (2014): 2439.
74. Mark Berman, Brady Dennis, and Elahe Izadi, "First U.S. Case of Ebola Diagnosed in Texas after Man Who Came from Liberia Falls Ill," *Washington Post*, September 30, 2014, http://www.washingtonpost.com/national/health-science/2014/09/30/2690947e-48f3-11e4-a046-120a8a855cca_story.html.
75. "The Ebola Alarmists," *Economist*, October 11, 2014, http://www.economist.com/news/united-states/21623713-stoking-panic-will-not-help-america-fight-ebola-ebola-alarmists.
76. Chad Livengood, "Land Urges Travel Ban to Ebola-Stricken Nations," *Detroit News*, October 3, 2014, http://www.detroitnews.com/story/news/politics/2014/10/03/terri-lynn-land-urges-travel-ban-ebola/16648683/.
77. Centers for Disease Control and Prevention, "Enhanced Ebola Screening to Start at Five U.S. Airports and New Tracking Program for all People Entering U.S. from Ebola-affected Countries," October 8, 2014, http://www.cdc.gov/media/releases/2014/p1008-ebola-screening.html.
78. "Ebola Outbreak: New York Doctor Craig Spencer Tests Positive," BBC News, October 24, 2014, http://www.bbc.co.uk/news/world-us-canada-29751495.
79. Kate Zernike and Thomas Kaplan, "Two Governors' Shifts on Ebola Are Criticized as Politics, Not Science," *New York Times*, October 28, 2014, A13.
80. Mark Berman, "New York, New Jersey, and Illinois to Quarantine Medical Workers Returning from West Africa," *Washington Post*, October 24, 2014, http://www.washingtonpost.com/news/post-nation/wp/2014/10/24/new-york-new-jersey-to-quarantine-medical-workers-returning-from-west-africa/ (accessed May 28, 2015).
81. Gregg Gonsalves and Peter Staley, "Panic, Paranoia, and Public Health—The AIDS Epidemic's Lessons for Ebola," *New England Journal of Medicine* 371, no. 25 (December 18, 2014): 2348.
82. Chris Jansing, "Samantha Power Travels to Guinea amid Ebola Outbreak," NBC News, October 21, 2014, http://www.nbcnews.com/storyline/ebola-virus-outbreak/samantha-power-travels-guinea-amid-ebola-outbreak-n234081. See also Lauren Gambino, "Ebola Nurse 'Made to Feel Like Criminal' on Return to US," *Guardian* (London), October 25, 2014, http://www.theguardian.com/world/2014/oct/25/obama-facts-not-fear-public-response-ebola-usa.
83. Paul Waldman, "Americans Are Terrified of Ebola, Which Could Make It Harder to Stop Ebola," *Washington Post*, October 14, 2014, http://www.washington post.com/blogs/plum-line/wp/2014/10/14/americans-are-terrified-of-ebola-which-could-make-it-harder-to-stop-ebola/.
84. Kelley Lee and David P. Fidler, "Avian and Pandemic Influenza: Progress and Problems with Global Health Governance," *Global Public Health* 2, no. 3 (2007): 226.
85. Julia Medew, "Airports to Screen All Passengers Entering Australia for Swine Flu," Traveller website (Fairfax Media), April 30, 2009, http://www.traveller.com.au/airports-to-screen-all-passengers-entering-australia-for-swine-flu-ao7v.

86. Brian Knowlton, "Two Flights Carried Man with Deadly TB," *New York Times*, May 29, 2007, http://www.nytimes.com/2007/05/29/health/29cnd-tb.html.

87. See Manny Fernandez, "Ebola Crisis Brings an Abundance of Caution into a Dallas Community," *New York Times*, October 4, 2014, A13; Tara Kirk Sell and Crystal Boddie, "'Out of an Abundance of Caution'—An Overused Phrase," *Bifurcated Needle*, July 22, 2015, http://www.bifurcatedneedle.com/new-blog/2015/7/22/out-of-an-abundance-of-caution-an-overused-phrase.

PART IV

ATTENTION OR NEGLECT

7

THE AGENDA OF GLOBAL HEALTH SECURITY

IN EARLY 2015 the US Presidential Commission for the Study of Bioethical Issues inquired into the ethical challenges arising from the Ebola outbreak then ongoing in West Africa. At a meeting with members of the commission, epidemiologist William Foege observed:

> All through medical training, you keep hearing the words "do no harm" . . . [but] you kill far more people, cause far more damage by the things you don't do, by the science that you don't apply, the science you don't share, the vaccines you don't use, the inequities that you don't pursue. I think that the single biggest biomedical ethical battleground of today is found in budgets.[1]

Foege's observation highlights the harmful neglect that can sometimes result from prioritizing attention to certain health issues over others. With regard to infectious diseases, an "attention or neglect" dilemma can arise from a government's efforts to reduce the risk of a dreaded germ emerging in its national territory. Such risk reduction can take the form of border controls or laboratory regulations. However, the practice of biosecurity can also manifest more generally in national and international policy settings in public health systems that systematically prioritize a narrow range of infectious disease risks. The ethical concern here, as with the other three kinds of biosecurity dilemma already discussed, is that a security-oriented approach should achieve more benefit than harm. Specifically, when it comes to setting priorities and allocating resources, the policy challenge is somehow to achieve extra protection against outbreaks of dreaded diseases, including diseases of biological weapons concern, without neglecting and perhaps thereby worsening other public health problems over the long term.

Broadly speaking, the tension at the heart of the attention or neglect biosecurity dilemma lies between policy approaches that might satisfy the greatest quantum of human need versus those that are politically feasible. On the one hand, a security-oriented approach to disease risks might succeed in improving the protection of human health, but only to the extent that a direct and immediate connection to national interest could plausibly be drawn. On the other hand, an approach that instead has a broadly humanitarian rationale might promise better health for many more people, but it might fail to receive political (and financial) support over a long enough period of time. In chapter 8 the problem of how to justly prioritize effort and allocate resources at the national level will be considered; in the US context, a biosecurity dilemma can arise from policy focused on domestic capacity to resist biological attacks. The task of the present chapter is to explore the attention or neglect dilemma in reference to "global health security" as an international-level biosecurity practice. As a practice that is essentially cooperative, it stands in contrast to the divisiveness of international bordering discussed earlier. At the same time, as the discussion will show, the shaping and pursuit of an agenda of global health security can be closely connected to national self-interest.

This chapter provides first an overview of the global health security agenda, currently being pursued most conspicuously by the WHO and the US government, that emphasizes surveillance of and rapid response to deadly and contagious infectious diseases. Although this "global" agenda tends toward protecting populations in developed states rather than promoting good health on a universal basis, it nevertheless has the potential to bring about an overall improvement in worldwide public health. This chapter discusses the capacity to respond rapidly to "public health emergencies of international concern" (PHEICs), and in so doing it extends the previous two chapters' assessment of the 2014 Ebola outbreak in West Africa. Beyond the remedy or overkill dilemma associated with social distancing and border security, the emergency-mode response to that outbreak also highlights the dynamics of attention and neglect at work in international, security-oriented health governance arrangements. Finally, the chapter considers surveillance for pandemic influenza as a dimension of global health security. The principal benefit of global influenza surveillance is supposed to be the affording of an early warning to all of the emergence of a pandemic virus anywhere in the world. However, the value of such warning is potentially diminished by the continued inability of many countries to secure an adequate supply of pandemic influenza vaccines.

INFECTIOUS DISEASES AND GLOBAL HEALTH SECURITY

The term "global health" implies consideration of the health of all people everywhere, as distinct from consideration of the health of people only within a particular community (e.g., nation or state). That which is "global" is arguably all-encompassing, and yet the policies and practices that purport to address global health problems tend to be selective in one way or another when it comes to expending effort and allocating resources. To illustrate this, David Stuckler and Martin McKee have identified a number of "metaphors" for global health used by policymakers. One of these is "global health as security," according to which "health policy seeks to protect one's own [national] population, focusing mainly on communicable diseases that threaten this population."[2] This may be contrasted with the metaphor of "global health as public health," where resources are directed toward "decreas[ing] the worldwide burden of disease, with priority given to those risk factors and diseases that make the greatest contribution to this burden."[3] Both approaches necessarily involve affording greater attention to some diseases and some people to the relative neglect of others. Neglect per se is inevitable whenever there is not equal and constant attention by everyone to all issues of (and related to) human health. That which may be the subject of political disagreement is really the particular *degree* to which certain diseases and people are apparently prioritized or neglected. Prioritization in the name of "security" can be especially controversial in matters of health policy, as can be seen in some of the advantages and disadvantages that result from the contemporary agenda of global health security. Even if it is focused mainly on the diseases that inspire dread in developed countries, could such an agenda also satisfy health needs in developed and developing countries alike? Or is the practice of global health security so excessively attentive to addressing particular infectious disease risks in particular ways that it neglects other important health issues?

It is worth recalling that "global health," as a discipline of medical science, is the sociotechnical descendent of what was previously called "colonial," "imperial," or "tropical" medicine.[4] A security element was already discernible in the latter label in the sense that, in Europe in the nineteenth century, referring to parts of the world as "the tropics" was "a way for imperial powers to define something culturally alien to, environmentally distinct from, and even threatening to Europe and other temperate regions."[5] In accordance with this view, as Scott Watson has observed, the discourse and practice of "tropical" medicine effectively "defined large portions of the earth as zones of danger for Europeans."[6] Thus, insofar as a legacy of power and differentiation informs global health as the disciplinary successor to tropical medicine, it should not come as a surprise that "global health *security*" is in practice focused on "the protection of the West from threats emanating from the developing world."[7] These "threats" are deadly infectious diseases of a kind which, until relatively recently, were generally thought to be in decline. Cholera, which originally emanated from South Asia, had for a long time threatened the health of populations in nineteenth-century Europe, but sanitation and other public health improvements soon reduced the incidence of this disease. Other diseases were resisted in like fashion, and advances in vaccine and antibiotic technology during the twentieth century served to further decrease the burden of infection in industrially advanced countries. For a time there was even some optimism in the West that people and policymakers could soon forget about microorganisms entirely as a source of disease.

This optimism eventually faltered as globalization gathered pace, bringing all the people of the world (and the microbes within their bodies) into closer and more constant contact. By the late twentieth century, deadly infectious diseases seemed again to be on the march, generating national and international concern for public health and security. In a 1992 report titled *Emerging Infections: Microbial Threats to Health in the United States*, the US Institute of Medicine warned that "some infectious diseases that now affect people in other parts of the world represent potential threats to the United States because of global interdependence."[8] In 1996 the World Health Report included an observation by WHO director-general Hiroshi Nakajima: "We are standing on the brink of a global crisis of infectious diseases. No country is safe from them. No country can any longer afford to ignore their threat."[9] Both of these predictions of impending or "emergent" microbial disaster framed infectious diseases as a matter of urgent political concern, and afterward both the US government and the WHO went so far as to resort to the language of security. Since the turn of the millennium each has pursued largely similar agendas of "global health security," but these have not been aimed at securing *everyone* against *all* health risks. Rather, in principle and in practice, securing global health has mainly been a project of developing and maintaining a strong capacity for detecting and responding only to certain kinds of infectious disease risks.

At the time of the anthrax attacks in the United States in late 2001—which reinforced the view among US and WHO policymakers that some pathogenic microorganisms should be framed in security terms—the shaping of a global health security agenda focused on infectious disease risks was already under way. In 2000 a declassified report by the US National Intelligence Council titled *The Global Infectious Disease Threat and Its Implications for the United States* warned: "New and reemerging infectious diseases will pose a rising global health threat and will complicate US and global security over the next 20 years."[10] At the WHA of May 2001, Resolution 54.14 (titled *Global Health Security: Epidemic Alert and Response*) recognized that "any upsurge in cases of infectious disease in a given country is potentially of concern for the international community."[11] The Resolution urged WHO member states to "participate actively in the verification and validation of surveillance data and information concerning health emergencies of international concern" and to "develop and update national preparation and response plans."[12] By the end of that year, and in response to the aforementioned anthrax attacks, the WHA's term "global health security" had also been adopted through a new Global Health Security Initiative (GHSI). Launched in November 2001, the GHSI is an informal arrangement involving Canada, France, Germany, Italy, Japan, Mexico, the United States, the United Kingdom, and the European Commission, with the WHO acting as an observer. Initially the participants framed global health security narrowly and called only for "concerted global action to strengthen public health preparedness and response to the threat of international biological, chemical and radio-nuclear terrorism," although in 2002 they broadened the scope of the initiative to include pandemic influenza.[13]

Meanwhile, the WHO itself maintained a broader frame for discussing global health security, which was consistent with WHA Resolution 54.14. In 2003 this broader view was vindicated with the outbreak of SARS. That outbreak made clear that, beyond the public health effects of bioterrorism and pandemic influenza, new infectious diseases that are contagious and deadly could constitute what the resolution had termed "health emergencies of international concern." Thus, SARS served to accelerate political efforts to draft and promulgate new IHRs, which the WHO later described as "an instrument of global public health security."[14] In 1995, following an Ebola outbreak in the Democratic Republic of Congo, the WHA had resolved to revise the 1969 IHRs. At the time of that outbreak (and in 2003, when SARS was spreading), the regulations required WHO member states to report outbreaks of only three diseases (cholera, plague, and yellow fever). To address the concern that the emergence and spread of deadly pathogens was outpacing international law, revisions to the IHRs agreed to in 2005 were designed to cover any infectious disease outbreak that fulfilled broad criteria for a "public health emergency of international concern" (PHEIC). As a result, the IHRs now place states under a legal obligation to (1) report these types of outbreak quickly to the WHO and (2) maintain their own core capacities for disease surveillance and rapid response. According to the WHO, in this way the IHRs amount to "a strategy of proactive risk management" that "aims to detect an [outbreak] event and stop it at its source—before it has a chance to become an international threat."[15]

GLOBAL HEALTH SECURITY AS A BIOSECURITY PRACTICE

Under Article 6 of the IHR every WHO member state must notify the WHO, within twenty-four hours of assessment of public health information, of all "events which may constitute a public health emergency of international concern within its territory." Such assessment is to occur by reference to a decision instrument in annex 2 of the regulations. Four diseases are automatically notifiable: smallpox, polio, SARS, and any new subtype of human influenza. In addition, a PHEIC assessment must be conducted if cholera, pneumonic plague, yellow fever, a viral hemorrhagic fever (e.g., Ebola), West Nile fever, or any other disease "of special national or regional concern" is detected by a national disease surveillance system. The regulations provide four criteria to assist governments in deciding whether the WHO must be informed about an outbreak event: (1) Is the public health impact of the event serious? (2) Is the event unusual or unexpected? (3) Is there a significant risk of international spread? and (4) Is there a significant risk of international restrictions to travel and trade?[16] Closely related to this reporting obligation is the requirement for all WHO member states to establish and maintain a set of "core capacity requirements for surveillance and response" (annex 1). States must have the capacity, for example, to "assess all reports of urgent events within forty-eight hours" and to provide support on a twenty-four-hour basis for a public health response through "specialized staff, laboratory analysis of samples . . . and logistical assistance."[17] The WHO maintains a Global Outbreak Alert and Response Network, which is intended to provide timely reports of infectious disease outbreaks and comprises over one hundred laboratories and national disease-reporting systems. Ideally with these highly sensitive and well-connected systems for local disease surveillance in place, outbreaks of deadly and contagious diseases will be detected and potentially contained rapidly wherever in the world they occur. Developing countries with little or no disease surveillance capacity continue to be the weak links in this chain. Yet, inasmuch as the IHRs are supposed to be an "instrument of global public health security," it is worth noting that the regulations make no provision for poorer WHO member states to receive the material assistance they need in order to strengthen their disease surveillance and response systems.[18] This might partly explain why, as of June 2012 (the deadline for achieving full IHR compliance), only 42 out of 194 WHO member states had reported on their fulfillment of core capacity requirements.

In response to this shortfall in member states reporting, US president Barack Obama launched a US-led Global Health Security Agenda (GHSA) in February 2014 "to accelerate progress toward a world safe and secure from infectious disease threats and to promote global health security as an international security priority."[19] The GHSA, which the US government claimed would extend to thirty countries within five years (and cover 4 billion people) is aimed at enabling those countries to better prevent, detect, and respond to public health emergencies. The nine objectives of the agenda, which overlap with the core capacities specified in the IHRs, are

1. Prevent the emergence and spread of antimicrobial drug resistant organisms and emerging zoonotic [animal to human transmissible] diseases, and strengthen international regulatory frameworks governing food safety.
2. Promote national biosafety and biosecurity systems.
3. Reduce the number and magnitude of infectious disease outbreaks.
4. Launch, strengthen, and link global networks for real-time biosurveillance.
5. Strengthen the global norm of rapid, transparent reporting and sample sharing.
6. Develop and deploy novel diagnostics and strengthen laboratory systems.
7. Train and deploy an effective biosurveillance workforce.
8. Develop an interconnected global network of Emergency Operations Centers and multi-sectoral response to biological incidents.
9. Improve global access to medical and non-medical countermeasures during health emergencies.[20]

As of July 2015 the US government had committed to invest $1 billion in seventeen countries through the GHSA.[21] However, it is important to acknowledge that this was thereby also an investment in furthering stated US policy on *national* security. For example, the 2010 National Security Strategy states that "the United States has a . . . strategic interest in promoting global health."[22] The first objective of the 2009 National Strategy for Countering Biological Threats is to "promote global health security" by "building global capacity for disease surveillance, detection, diagnosis, and reporting" and "improving international capacity against infectious diseases."[23] One of the objectives of the 2015 National Health Security Strategy is to "strengthen global health security and, as a result, [America's] own health security" by "working . . . with international partners to develop global capacities and operational capabilities to prevent epidemics, detect threats early, rapidly respond to incidents, and support integrated recovery efforts."[24] US engagement with an agenda of global health security might thus be perceived merely as a global means to achieving a national end. Even so, such engagement apparently has the potential to generate at least some biosecurity benefits for those countries on the receiving end of the efforts, resources, and expertise of the United States.

One example of this double effect is the local benefit that was derived from a "GHS [global health security] demonstration project" conducted in Uganda in 2013. The project, which involved the CDC and the Uganda Ministry of Health, implemented improvements to local disease surveillance in three areas: (1) strengthening the public health laboratory system by increasing the capacity of diagnostic and specimen referral networks, (2) enhancing the existing communications and information systems for outbreak response, and (3) developing a public health emergency operations center. For indicators to assess enhancements made through implementation of the project, the Ugandan government selected three "priority pathogens" that (in Uganda) were deemed most likely to generate a PHEIC: multidrug-resistant *Mycobacterium tuberculosis* (TB), *Vibrio cholerae* (cholera), and the Ebola virus. One of the outcomes of the GHS demonstration project was the "development of an outbreak response module that allowed reporting of suspected cases of illness caused by priority pathogens via . . . SMS [short message service] . . . to the Uganda District Health Information System." Another was the "expansion of the biologic specimen transport and laboratory reporting system supported by the [US] President's Emergency Plan for AIDS Relief."[25]

For present purposes, the selection of specific diseases (MDR-TB, cholera, and Ebola) to be included in this US-sponsored project is significant, as is the public health burden that each disease poses locally. The WHO counts Uganda among twenty-two "high burden countries" for TB but not for MDR-TB, and in 2013 only an estimated 1.4 percent of TB cases were multidrug resistant.[26] Between 1997 and 2010 an estimated average of 11,000 cholera cases (including between 61 and 182 deaths) occurred in Uganda each year.[27] Prior to 2014 the largest-ever Ebola outbreak had occurred in Uganda in 2000–2001 (resulting in 224 deaths out of 425 cases), and smaller outbreaks had also occurred there in 2007, 2011, and 2012.[28] Clearly the burden posed by these three diseases was real when they received attention from the US and Ugandan governments in the name of "global health security." However, a question that arises from a humanitarian perspective is whether such attention might on this occasion have been more fruitfully directed elsewhere. That is, could more lives have been saved, prolonged, or improved if other diseases or health issues had instead been addressed? It is worth noting that in Uganda in 2013 (when the CDC's demonstration project was conducted) there were, for example, over 1.5 million reported cases of malaria (including 7,277 deaths) and the maternal mortality rate was 360 per 100,000 population.[29] Moreover, according to the most recent WHO data, Uganda contains only 0.117 physicians per 1,000 population (compared to 2.452 in the United States), which reflects a broader problem of health system weakness.[30]

Attention or Neglect?

The Uganda example illustrates the potential for global health security, as a biosecurity practice, to give rise to an attention or neglect dilemma. On the one hand, a disease surveillance improvement project focused on "priority pathogens" (which cause dreaded diseases) was obviously a politically feasible one from the US government's perspective. The project furthered the objectives of US national security policy as well as the IHRs, and it also provided some local benefit. On the other hand, a greater quantum of health need in Uganda might have been fulfilled had more burdensome diseases or the Ugandan health system generally received an equal measure of attention. It seems less likely that the latter option would have attracted the necessary long-term political (and financial) support. For better or for worse, in the sphere of public health and elsewhere, political action driven by a concern for security is often more likely and more powerful than action driven by other (e.g., humanitarian) concerns. This is probably why, in 2007, the WHO elected to "play the security card" with regard to global health.[31]

In the year when the revised IHRs entered into force, the WHO's annual World Health Report defined "global public health security" as "the activities required, both proactive and reactive, to minimize vulnerability to acute public health events that endanger the collective health of populations living across geographical regions and international boundaries."[32] The implication of such framing, however, was that problems of a non-"acute" nature were excluded from the organization's global health security agenda, even though the sum of such problems accounts for the greater part of health need throughout the world. For this reason the institutionalized privileging of certain disease risks with security status has been the subject of much lamentation. In the academic literature focused on the linking of health and security, a common refrain has been that biological attacks and other dreaded disease risks receive too much attention and that, consequently, other health burdens (as reflected in disease statistics) are neglected. For example, Colleen O'Manique has claimed that "today's health and security agenda ignores . . . the boring, persistent, communicable and non-communicable diseases that in fact kill more people annually worldwide than high-profile diseases."[33] Alexander Kelle observed in 2007 that the IHR definition of PHEICs "appears to be much more oriented toward the US Center for Disease Control's list of bioterrorism [select] agents than those disease-causing agents that have caused the most fatalities over the last decade."[34] Along similar lines, Debra DeLaet has argued that "the process by which some diseases are securitized and others are not" is driven by "the political interests, strategic calculations, and influence of key actors in global health rather than a reflection of an objective assessment of where the most critical health needs exist."[35]

The suggestion by these and other analysts seems to be that more lives would be saved, and a greater quantum of health need fulfilled, if political attention were diverted away from diseases deemed to be of security concern and redirected toward those health risks that are presently "the real killers." Such an argument resonates strongly with the aforementioned metaphor of "global health as public health," according to which effort and resources are devoted to maximizing the overall reduction of present (and thus measurable) health burdens. However, as an example of "objective utilitarianism" (a concept explored in the next chapter), this approach is fundamentally challenged by at least one nonobjective factor: the fear of *future* infectious disease outbreaks that would impose a burden that is presently unmeasurable. Across time, the inherent difficulty of balancing the measurable against the unmeasurable compounds the attention or neglect dilemma, even though the appropriate prioritization of effort and resources might seem obvious at a given *moment* in time. It is not enough at that moment to assemble health statistics demonstrating the actual burden of various disease risks and to contrast this burden with the nonoccurrence of, say, an influenza pandemic or a biological attack. Any priority-setting that is based solely on such an assessment would fail thereafter to account for the possibility that the future might differ from the present. From the perspective of governments in developing countries, preparing for future "acute public health events" might appear, in the present, to entail neglecting serious health burdens of an ongoing nature.[36] However, it could also be argued that those governments have a long-term interest in playing along with developed countries' desire to strengthen disease surveillance and response capacity worldwide. Poorer populations are, after all, generally more vulnerable to the effects of transnational epidemics when they eventually occur.[37]

To assess the notion that the agenda of global health security works to the advantage of developed and developing countries alike, the sections that follow consider rapid international responses to PHEICs and worldwide disease surveillance with regard to Ebola and pandemic influenza, respectively. In each instance the concern is whether institutionalized governance arrangements enabling immediate attention to an emerging and dreaded disease risk also have the potential to perpetuate the neglect of other health-relevant problems.

The Emergency Response to Ebola in West Africa

The Ebola outbreak in West Africa that began in early 2014 ended up causing illness and death on a relatively small scale. At the time of writing, the WHO was reporting a worldwide total of 11,316 deaths from among 28,639 confirmed cases of Ebola, almost all of them occurring in Guinea, Liberia, and Sierra Leone.[38] Even taking into account the probably large number of unreported cases, on this occasion Ebola exacted a health toll far less than that exacted on an ongoing basis by other diseases prevalent in that part of the world (such as HIV/AIDS, malaria, and TB). While it would be neither helpful nor fair to make a judgment in hindsight that the Ebola outbreak as a whole received excessive attention, it does matter that when the WHO declared the outbreak to be a PHEIC on August 8, 2014, there was a high degree of political and popular concern at the time that the disease *might* spread much further and kill many more people than it did. Framing the Ebola outbreak as an emergency in IHR terms afforded political space for the implementation of extraordinary response measures. These measures included quarantine zones and travel restrictions imposed unilaterally by individual states. In addition, the Ebola outbreak occasioned states to respond in emergency mode on a collective basis under WHO and US leadership. It is worth considering, then, the advantages and disadvantages of attending to this disease as a matter of global health security. On the one hand, the international-level emergency response to Ebola was apparently highly effective at containing the outbreak. On the other, it might have established a precedent for responding in like fashion again while neglecting over time the local health conditions that likely caused and prolonged the outbreak.

On the same day that the UN Security Council described the Ebola outbreak as "a threat to international peace and security," UN secretary-general Ban Ki-moon announced his decision to establish a UN Mission for Ebola Emergency Response (UNMEER).[39] He claimed, "This unprecedented situation requires unprecedented steps to save lives and safeguard peace and security."[40] The establishment of UNMEER was unanimously endorsed by UN member states through General Assembly Resolution 69/1, and the mission operated from September 19, 2014, through July 31, 2015.[41] The resolution's core objective was to scale up the on-the-ground response to Ebola and to establish unity of purpose among all responders in support of locally led disease control efforts. To that end, UNMEER channeled financial, logistical, and human resources to Guinea, Liberia, and Sierra Leone with a view to achieving zero cases of Ebola in those three countries.[42] The scale and swiftness of this enterprise, its instigation by the UN secretary-general (rather than by the WHO director-general), and the fact that it was called a "mission" (a UN term that normally refers to peacekeeping operations) were extraordinary characteristics of the international response to Ebola. In addition, a salient aspect of that response was the use of military resources for disease-control purposes.

In September 2014, when it appeared that the situation in West Africa would very soon worsen precipitously, the US government placed itself at the forefront of international efforts to bring Ebola under control. On September 16 President Obama announced plans to send as many as three thousand US military personnel, headquartered in Liberia, to build as many as seventeen Ebola treatment centers (each with one hundred beds) in affected areas of West Africa.[43] Britain and France followed, directing similar but smaller military commitments to Sierra Leone and Guinea, respectively.[44] Resolution 2177 from the UN Security Council welcomed "the support of the defence forces" of African Union states toward containing the spread of Ebola.[45] Obama, in explaining his decision, described the Ebola outbreak as "a potential threat to global security."[46] Against this threat, US forces were to bring "expertise in command and control, in logistics, in engineering," and the president boasted: "Our Armed Services are better at that than any organization on Earth."[47] The obvious advantage of deploying advanced military capabilities to help control a disease outbreak is that it can be done quickly and on a large scale. Even so, this advantage could only be achieved by a given military organization if its capabilities were not needed or already being used elsewhere. As such, although military resources were in fact able to be used against Ebola in West Africa in 2014, it might be difficult in practice to rely *generally* on the availability of a military response for disease-control purposes.

In addition, incorporating a military dimension into the response to an outbreak might also be a bad idea in principle. Alex de Waal has argued, for example, that military involvement in the response to Ebola in West Africa was "worryingly authoritarian, bad for public health, and strategically counterproductive."[48] In his view, despite an army's "impressive logistics," soldiers' participation in disaster relief often makes things worse:

> they utilize vast amounts of oversized equipment, clogging up scarce airport facilities, docks and roads; their heavy machinery damages local infrastructure; they use more equipment and personnel in building their own bases and protecting themselves than in doing the job; [and] their militarized attitudes offend local sensibilities and generate resentment.[49]

To the extent that this characterization is true, the devotion of military-based attention to the Ebola outbreak might well have been partly counterproductive, and the last of de Waal's allegations is of particular concern from a public health perspective. In Guinea, Liberia, and Sierra Leone, which in 2014 had only recently emerged from years of civil conflict, people's trust in government (which is essential for disease-control purposes) was difficult to maintain, especially when the government deployed its military. Thus it seems reasonable to suggest that the presence of *foreign* troops might have compounded rather than reduced the problem of maintaining public trust. More generally, according to Melissa Leach, the lesson of previous Ebola outbreaks has been that local populations tend to have "a broader distrust of international teams 'parachuted' in from outside."[50] Indeed, when outsiders appear suddenly and act hastily in the midst of a disease outbreak, it might be difficult initially to accept that their actions are genuinely well intended. If, for example, little or no external assistance has been forthcoming with regard to serious and ongoing illnesses experienced by a local community, a sudden international concern to address one particular disease might appear suspicious. As Ranu Dhillon and Daniel Kelly have observed, when local people "cannot find care for a child with diarrheal disease, they question the sincerity of response teams that seem eager to help them with Ebola."[51]

Over the long term the problem with relying mainly on emergency-mode responses (military or otherwise) to PHEICs might be that global health security becomes merely a process of constantly managing disease crises in the developing world. This can be contrasted with a response mode that additionally emphasizes improving health system capabilities in areas prone to outbreaks. One of the major lessons of the Ebola outbreak in West Africa was that better public health conditions there would have made contagion less extensive. In Guinea, Liberia, and Sierra Leone, too few qualified health workers were locally available at the time, and health services were poorly organized and managed. Government expenditure on health was low, and there were ongoing logistical, disease surveillance, and drug supply problems.[52] Accordingly, the WHO argued in a 2015 planning document that "Ebola became epidemic in the affected areas in large part because of the weakness of the health systems."[53] Nevertheless, by the time the outbreak was slowing down, the prevailing view within the WHO hierarchy appeared to be that emergency-mode responses should still be emphasized over preventive (system-strengthening) action.

In April 2015, in a statement on the Ebola response that detailed a number of "learned lessons," the organization's senior officials called on national governments to "take disease threats seriously."[54] This was to be done by "investing . . . in essential public health systems for preparedness, surveillance and response, which are fully integrated and aligned with efforts to strengthen health systems." However, the statement envisaged no specific mechanisms for assisting poorer countries to make such an investment. By contrast, the WHO leadership announced the creation of a global health emergency workforce consisting of "teams of trained and certified responders who can be available immediately" and of a contingency fund to enable the organization to "respond more rapidly to disease outbreaks."[55] In thus reserving expertise and resources for a "rainy day," though, the WHO effectively prevented these from being used in outbreak-prone areas of the world on an everyday basis. Attention was once again directed mainly toward short-term responses to future disease risks with international reach and the need for ongoing strengthening of poor countries' health systems remained relatively neglected.

Surveillance and Vaccines for Pandemic Influenza

Neglect of systemic problems is apparent also with regard to pandemic influenza, even though that disease is afforded priority attention as a matter of global health security. Under the IHRs, a new subtype of human influenza is automatically notifiable to the WHO which, in 2007, described pandemic influenza as "the most feared security threat."[56] The principal benefit to be derived from global surveillance of influenza viruses is an early warning to all governments of the emergence of a virus with pandemic properties. Such warning of the commencement of human-to-human viral transmission is valuable because it allows everyone more time to organize and implement a response. To that extent, disease surveillance may be regarded as a global public good.[57] The response could be of a nonpharmaceutical kind but could give rise to a remedy or overkill dilemma. Therefore, in order to minimize the damage and disruption caused by social distancing, governments generally prefer to protect their populations through vaccination against pandemic influenza. The problem that presently exists, however, is that the total amount of influenza vaccine able to be produced annually is nowhere near enough to protect everyone everywhere. In other words, the availability of a pandemic vaccine is not truly global, despite pandemic influenza having acquired priority status as a dreaded disease that poses a global health security risk. Only the wealthiest of countries, where governments have preordered doses of vaccine, are able to take full advantage of influenza surveillance as a global biosecurity practice.

Based on current technology, the development and production of a vaccine matched to a pandemic virus can commence only once that virus has started spreading. The standard decades-old method of producing influenza vaccines is to grow virus inside hens' eggs, and it typically takes several months for doses to become available. These are then delivered to countries that are best able to pay and in which the major producers of influenza vaccine operate. In June 2009, for example, the United States had already ordered 40 million doses of vaccine against swine flu, the United Kingdom 90 million, and France 50 million.[58] Six months into that pandemic, only 534 million doses were available worldwide, and after one year there were 1.3 billion.[59] Thus, for the duration of the pandemic, a large majority of the world's population of nearly seven billion people remained unprotected by vaccination. Fortunately, the swine flu pandemic turned out to be a mild one. Nevertheless, concerns about vaccine availability had earlier been raised by some developing countries with regard to another disease with pandemic potential: H5N1 bird flu. The Indonesian government in particular drew attention to its concerns by withholding samples of H5N1 virus from the WHO Global Influenza Surveillance Network.

When Indonesia suddenly withdrew from the network in January 2007, it was continuing to experience many more human H5N1 cases than any other country. As such, Indonesia was the most important source of information on that virus's properties and whether it might be mutating into a pandemic form. From this position of "strength," Indonesian health minister Siti Supari applied political pressure in furtherance of what she perceived as her country's national interest. She first accused the WHO of transferring viral samples of Indonesian origin to pharmaceutical companies to make influenza vaccines for which the Indonesian people would have to pay an unacceptably high price. Supari then reportedly agreed to supply H5N1 samples directly to the US-based company Baxter Healthcare, with a view to securing an affordable pandemic vaccine in the future.[60] Later, at a meeting with WHO officials in March 2007, Supari sought assurances that Indonesia would get a vaccine if a pandemic occurred, and she described the global vaccine supply scheme then in place as "more dangerous than the threat of an H5N1 pandemic itself."[61] Against this backdrop, WHO assistant director-general David Heymann argued that "Indonesia is putting the public health security of the whole world at risk because they're not sharing [influenza] viruses."[62] What Indonesia was essentially claiming, though, was that poorer countries were already experiencing a high degree of insecurity and that cooperation with influenza researchers worldwide was pointless if those countries were unable to benefit from the vaccines that result from that cooperation. This claim presented a fundamental challenge to a notion at the core of the global health security agenda: that global disease surveillance is a governance arrangement that serves *local* public health needs.

In formal recognition of the concern represented by Indonesia's drastic action, the sixtieth WHA in May 2007 passed a resolution requesting the WHO to establish "an international stockpile of vaccines for H5N1 or other influenza viruses of pandemic potential" and to "formulate mechanisms and guidelines aimed at ensuring fair and equitable distribution of pandemic influenza vaccines at affordable prices in the event of a pandemic."[63] Four years later the WHA adopted the Pandemic Influenza Preparedness Framework [PIPF] for the Sharing of Influenza Viruses and Access to Vaccines and Other Benefits. The principles of the framework include recognition by WHO member states that "the benefits arising from the sharing of H5N1 and other influenza viruses with human pandemic potential should be shared" and that "global influenza vaccine production capacity remains insufficient to meet anticipated need in a pandemic."[64] There is recognition also of the need for "financing mechanisms that would promote affordability and equitable access to quality influenza vaccines . . . by developing countries."[65] For present purposes, however, it is significant that the PIPF is legally nonbinding, in contrast to the IHRs, which support the agenda of global health security. Whereas the key provisions of the latter (surveillance, reporting, and rapid response) have the status of international law, the PIPF merely urges WHO member states to perform certain actions and makes the desired increase in vaccine supplies almost entirely dependent on the voluntary cooperation and material generosity of nonstate actors (vaccine manufacturing companies). For example, the framework provides that "Member States should urge vaccine manufacturers to set aside a portion of each production cycle of pandemic influenza vaccine for use by developing countries."[66] As such, and despite the growing degree of political attention to the issue of global pandemic influenza vaccine supplies, the framework could also be characterized as an instrument for systematically denying the issue a place on the agenda of global health security. If it is, and if some countries perceive the continuation of a gap between disease surveillance expectations and public health benefits, the potential for another virus-sharing dispute remains.

CONCLUSION

In international policy settings for public health, priority attention and greater resources are always in some way directed toward some health issues to the relative neglect of others. The agenda of global health security, embodied by the WHO's IHRs and reinforced by the US-led GHSA, focuses mainly on surveillance of and rapid response to outbreaks of deadly and contagious diseases. To the extent that such outbreaks are likely to originate in poorer parts of the world, the agenda arguably resembles the bygone enterprise of "tropical medicine" aimed at protecting populations within Europe from infectious diseases without. A critical difference, though, is that the pursuit of a strong worldwide capacity for disease surveillance and response promises immediate benefits to developed and developing countries alike in the event of an outbreak with transnational reach. Even so, prioritizing political attention to this capacity has the potential also to perpetuate the neglect of other health-relevant problems that exist mainly in the developing world. That is, global health security as a biosecurity practice can give rise to an attention or neglect dilemma. Over the long term, the challenge for well-resourced policymakers in the developed world is to achieve greater protection of fearful populations against suddenly emerging PHEICs in a way that does not neglect ongoing health problems. Not least this is because such neglect has the potential to undermine international enthusiasm for and commitment to an agenda of global health security.

From the perspective of countries that are unlikely to access enough vaccines during an influenza pandemic, it might be difficult to reconcile the requirement for worldwide virus surveillance with the persistence of a vaccine supply system that benefits only a small minority of the world's population. A question that arises is, If pandemic influenza is a *global* health security risk, why is a critical pharmaceutical response not globally available? Although the 2011 PIPF goes some way to assuaging any such concerns, this nonbinding agreement among WHO member states is inherently less influential than the IHR. Thus, whereas surveillance and rapid response are prioritized via the agenda of global health security, the issue of pandemic influenza vaccine availability remains relatively and systematically neglected. Similarly, in the case of the 2014 Ebola outbreak in West Africa, global health security as a biosecurity practice demonstrated its potential to sideline the remedying of underlying health problems and inequities. One lesson from that outbreak is that appealing to global security, as President Obama did, can be valuable as a spur to public health action. Indeed, the political attention afforded to Ebola as a matter of global health security was apparently beneficial in the short term. The public profile of the disease was thereby raised, abundant resources were made available, and a large-scale international project of disease-control was swiftly established. This success might even have suggested to WHO and national government leaders that they could respond in like fashion again, thus entrenching the place of rapid response on the agenda of global health security. However, in contrast to the maintenance of a posture of preparedness to engage in time-critical crisis management, a long-term response to Ebola in Africa is arguably more likely to be found in ongoing improvement of the structural and socioeconomic conditions that currently pose a more general risk to public health.

Although the apparent disparity between global health needs and global health security priorities can at times seem irrational, the attention or neglect dilemma cannot be avoided simply by affording the greatest degree of attention to risks that presently pose the greatest health burden worldwide from year to year. To do so would only perpetuate neglect of the future risk and possibly the heavy health burden of some kinds of outbreak events. Rather, this biosecurity dilemma presents the vexing challenge of somehow maximizing the fulfillment of human need within the shifting bounds of political feasibility. At present, a particular agenda of global health security is politically strengthened by its explicit alignment with the national security interests of the United States, a country with vast scientific resources and expertise deployed in numerous other countries. If that agenda were less security-oriented and more broadly humanitarian in scope, however, it might fail to receive as much political support and thus might enable the saving—over time and throughout the world—of comparatively fewer lives. Problems of attention and neglect arising from a security-oriented approach to public health can also arise at the level of national policy, and these are addressed in the next chapter's discussion of policy settings within the United States itself.

Of particular interest is the US government's prioritization of efforts to defend the US population against biological attacks. So the discussion now returns to biodefense.

NOTES

1. William Foege, "Public Health Perspectives on the Current Ebola Epidemic in Western Africa," Presidential Commission for the Study of Bioethical Issues, February 5, 2015, http://bioethics.gov/node/4591.
2. David Stuckler and Martin McKee, "Five Metaphors about Global-Health Policy," *The Lancet* 372 (July 12, 2008): 96.
3. Ibid.
4. See Andrew D. Pinto, Anne-Emanuelle Birn, and Ross E. G. Upshur, "The Context of Global Health Ethics," in *An Introduction to Global Health Ethics*, ed. Andrew D. Pinto and Ross E. G. Upshur (New York: Routledge, 2013), 12.
5. Anne-Emanuelle Birn, "From Plagues to Peoples: Health on the Modern Global/International Agenda," in *Ashgate Research Companion to the Globalization of Health*, ed. Ted Schrecker (Farnham, UK: Ashgate, 2012), 43.
6. Scott Watson, "Back Home, Safe and Sound: The Public and Private Production of Insecurity," *International Political Sociology* 5 (2011): 163.
7. Simon Rushton, "Global Health Security: Security for Whom? Security from What?," *Political Studies* 59, no. 4 (2011): 780. See also Lorna Weir, "Inventing Global Health Security, 1994–2005," in *Routledge Handbook of Global Health Security*, ed. Simon Rushton and Jeremy Youde (New York: Routledge, 2015), 27; Lawrence Gostin, "The International Health Regulations and Beyond," *The Lancet Infectious Diseases* 4, no. 10 (2004): 606; and Colin McInnes and Kelley Lee, "Health, Security, and Foreign Policy," *Review of International Studies* 32, no. 1 (2006): 11. In addition, as an anonymous reviewer has helpfully pointed out, the security of countries outside "the West" (like China) can also be threatened by diseases that spread from other developing countries.
8. Joshua Lederberg, Robert E. Shope, and Stanley C. Oaks Jr., eds., *Emerging Infections: Microbial Threats to Health in the United States* (Washington, DC: National Academies Press, 1992), v.
9. World Health Organization, *Fighting Disease, Fostering Development*, World Health Report 1996, v.
10. Federation of American Scientists, "The Global Infectious Disease Threat and Its Implications for the United States," National Intelligence Estimate 99-17D, US National Intelligence Council (January 2000), http://www.fas.org/irp/threat/nie99-17d.htm.
11. "Global Health Security: Epidemic Alert and Response" (WHA54.14), 54th World Health Assembly, May 21, 2001.
12. Ibid.
13. "GHSI Background," Global Health Security Initiative, n.d., http://www.ghsi.ca/english/background.asp (accessed October 22, 2015).
14. World Health Organization, *A Safer Future: Global Public Health Security in the Twenty-First Century*, World Health Report 2007, ix.

15. Ibid., vii.
16. World Health Organization, *International Health Regulations 2005*, 2nd ed. (Geneva: World Health Organization, 2008), 43–46.
17. Ibid., 41.
18. World Health Organization, *A Safer Future*, ix.
19. US Department of Health and Human Services, "Global Health Security," n.d., http://www.globalhealth.gov/global-health-topics/global-health-security/ (accessed October 22, 2015).
20. Centers for Disease Control and Prevention, "The Global Health Security Agenda," August 20, 2014, http://www.cdc.gov/globalhealth/security/ghsagenda.htm.
21. Office of the Press Secretary, the White House, "Fact Sheet: The Global Health Security Agenda," July 28, 2015, https://www.whitehouse.gov/the-press-office/2015/07/28/fact-sheet-global-health-security-agenda.
22. The White House, "National Security Strategy," May 2010, https://www.white-house.gov/sites/default/files/rss_viewer/national_security_strategy.pdf, 39.
23. National Security Council, "National Strategy for Countering Biological Threats," November 2009: https://www.whitehouse.gov/sites/default/files/National_Strategy_for_Countering_BioThreats.pdf, 6–7.
24. US Department of Health and Human Services, "National Health Security Strategy and Implementation Plan 2015-2018," February 13, 2015, http://www.phe.gov/Preparedness/planning/authority/nhss/Pages/strategy.aspx.
25. Jeff N. Borchert et al., "Rapidly Building Global Health Security Capacity—Uganda Demonstration Project, 2013,'" *Morbidity and Mortality Weekly Report* 63, no. 4 (2014): 73–76.
26. World Health Organization, *Global Tuberculosis Report 2014*, 143.
27. Godfrey Bwire et al., "The Burden of Cholera in Uganda," *PLoS Neglected Tropical Diseases* 7, no. 12 (December 2013), http://journals.plos.org/plosntds/article?id=10.1371/journal.pntd.0002545.
28. US Centers for Disease Control and Prevention, "Ebola Outbreaks 2000–2014," September 3, 2015, http://www.cdc.gov/vhf/ebola/outbreaks/history/summaries.html.
29. World Health Organization, "Uganda Statistics Summary (2002–Present)," n.d., http://apps.who.int/gho/data/node.country.country-UGA?lang=en (accessed September 4, 2015).
30. World Health Organization, "Density per 1000 Data by Country, 2015," http://apps.who.int/gho/data/node.main.A1444 (accessed September 4, 2015).
31. See Stefan Elbe, "Should Health Professionals Play the Global Health Security Card?," *The Lancet* 378 (July 16, 2011): 220–21.
32. World Health Organization, *A Safer Future*, 5.
33. Colleen O'Manique, "Global Health and the Human Security Agenda," in *Ashgate Research Companion to the Globalization of Health*, ed. Ted Schrecker (Farnham, UK: Ashgate, 2012), 167.
34. Alexander Kelle, "Securitization of International Public Health: Implications for Global Health Governance and the Biological Weapons Prohibition Regime," *Global Governance* 13 (2007): 230–31.
35. Debra L. DeLaet, "Whose Interests Is the Securitization of Health Serving?," in *Routledge Handbook of Global Health Security*, ed. Simon Rushton and Jeremy Youde

(New York: Routledge, 2015), 342. See also Harley Feldbaum, Preeti Patel, Egbert Sondorp, and Kelley Lee, "Global Health and National Security: The Need for Critical Engagement," *Medicine, Conflict and Survival* 22, no. 3 (2006): 196; Sara E. Davies, *Global Politics of Health* (Cambridge: Polity, 2010), 138; and Michael A. Stevenson and Michael Moran, "Health Security and the Distortion of the Global Health Agenda," in *Routledge Handbook of Global Health Security*, ed. Simon Rushton and Jeremy Youde (New York: Routledge, 2015).

36. World Health Organization, *A Safer Future*, 5.

37. See Thomas R. Frieden et al., "Safer Countries through Global Health Security," *The Lancet* 383 (March 1, 2014): 764.

38. World Health Organization, "Ebola Situation Reports," updated March 13, 2016, http://apps.who.int/ebola/ebola-situation-reports (accessed March 29, 2016).

39. United Nations, Report No. S/RES/2177, September 18, 2014 (New York: United Nations, 2014).

40. United Nations, Report No. S/PV.7268, September 18, 2014 (New York: United Nations, 2014), 3.

41. United Nations, Report No. A/RES/69/1, September 19, 2014 (New York: United Nations, 2014), 2.

42. United Nations, "UN Mission for Ebola Emergency Response (UNMEER)," 2015, http://ebolaresponse.un.org/un-mission-ebola-emergency-response-unmeer.

43. Helene Cooper, Michael D. Shear, and Denise Grady, "Obama to Call for Expansion of Ebola Fight," *New York Times*, September 16, 2014, A1.

44. Andrew Higgins, "European Leaders Scramble to Upgrade Response to Ebola Crisis," *New York Times*, October 9, 2014, A16.

45. United Nations, Report No. S/RES/2177, September 18, 2014 (New York: United Nations, 2014), 2.

46. "Obama Says Ebola Outbreak a 'Global Security Threat,'" BBC News, September 17, 2014, http://www.bbc.co.uk/news/world-us-canada-29231400.

47. Dan Lamothe, "Meet the New U.S. Military Force that Obama Is Deploying to Fight Ebola," *Washington Post*, September 16, 2014, https://www.washington post.com/news/checkpoint/wp/2014/09/16/meet-the-new-u-s-military-force -that-obama-is-deploying-to-fight-ebola/.

48. Alex de Waal, "Militarizing Global Health," *Boston Review*, November 11, 2014, http://bostonreview.net/world/alex-de-waal-militarizing-global-health-ebola.

49. Ibid.

50. Melissa Leach, "Time to Put Ebola in Context," *Bulletin of the World Health Organization* 88, no. 7 (2010): 489.

51. Ranu S. Dhillon and J. Daniel Kelly, "Community Trust and the Ebola Endgame," *New England Journal of Medicine* 373, no. 9 (2015): 788.

52. Marie-Paule Kieny, David B. Evans, Gerard Schmets, and Sowmya Kadandale, "Health-System Resilience: Reflections on the Ebola Crisis in Western Africa," *Bulletin of the World Health Organization* 92, no. 12 (2014): 850.

53. World Health Organization, *2015 WHO Strategic Response Plan: West Africa Ebola Outbreak*, 13.

54. World Health Organization, "WHO Leadership Statement on the Ebola Response and WHO Reforms," April 16, 2015, http://www.who.int/csr/disease/ebola/joint -statement-ebola/en/.

55. Ibid.
56. World Health Organization, *A Safer Future*, 45.
57. See Mark W. Zacher, "Global Epidemiological Surveillance: International Cooperation to Monitor Infectious Diseases," in *Global Public Goods: International Cooperation in the Twenty-First Century*, ed. Inge Kaul, Isabelle Grunberg, and Marc Stern (New York: Oxford University Press, 1999), 268–69.
58. Erika Check Hayden, "Avian Influenza Aided Readiness for Swine Flu," *Nature* 459 (June 11, 2009): 756.
59. Klaus Stöhr, "Ill Prepared for a Pandemic," *Nature* 507 (March 6, 2014): S20.
60. Zakki Hakim, "Indonesia to Trade Flu Virus for Vaccine," *Washington Post*, February 16, 2007, http://www.washingtonpost.com/wp-dyn/content/article/2007/02/16/AR2007021600685.html.
61. Dennis Normile, "Indonesia to Share Flu Samples Under New Terms," *Science* 316 (April 6, 2007): 37.
62. Robert Roos, "WHO: Indonesia's Withholding of Viruses Endangers World," Center for Infectious Disease Research and Policy, University of Minnesota, August 7, 2007, http://www.cidrap.umn.edu/news-perspective/2007/08/who-indonesias-withholding-viruses-endangers-world.
63. World Health Organization, "World Health Assembly Closes," May 23, 2007, http://www.who.int/mediacentre/news/releases/2007/wha02/en/.
64. World Health Organization, *Pandemic Influenza Preparedness Framework for the Sharing of Influenza Viruses and Access to Vaccines and Other Benefits*, 2011, 3–4.
65. Ibid., 5.
66. Ibid., 20.

8

PUBLIC HEALTH AND BIODEFENSE PRIORITIES

THE ATTENTION OR NEGLECT DILEMMA, hitherto discussed in regard to international health governance arrangements, can also arise at the level of national policy. The prioritization of effort and resources for biosecurity purposes must also be explored specifically in the context of the United States, where the main concern is the policy emphasis on protecting the US population against future biological attacks. Such emphasis has the potential upside of improving the protective capacity of the public health system, but the downside is that it could also occasion insufficient emphasis on other health risks and lifesaving measures. Although naturally occurring outbreaks of dreaded diseases (e.g., pandemic influenza) are also the subject of special attention from US policymakers, the dread inspired by the notion of malicious infection is particularly powerful in a country that endured a series of deadly anthrax attacks in 2001. Following those attacks, the US government quickly realized that the effect of the attacks (five Americans killed) could have been far worse had a pathogenic microorganism other than noncontagious *Bacillus anthracis* been used. From that point on, US policy emphasized the need to protect people against a contagious pathogen that could emerge today only as a result of human activity: *variola major* (the smallpox virus).

The WHO had confirmed the eradication of that virus from nature in 1980. Smallpox as a human disease ceased to exist, but WHO member states allowed *variola major* to continue to exist in two secure laboratories (one inside the United States and the other inside the former Soviet Union). Thereafter, any smallpox outbreak could result only from a problem of laboratory biosafety or biosecurity: leakage or theft of the virus from a place authorized or not authorized to store it. It later became apparent that the anthrax attacks of 2001 resulted from such a problem, but one of the US government's immediate concerns when these attacks occurred was to seek protection against another kind of biological attack that would generate a greater degree of damage. As D. A. Henderson, who led the worldwide campaign to eradicate smallpox, has recalled,

> emergency meetings were convened as we pondered threats and decided what should be given highest priority. There was no question but that smallpox virus as a biological weapon posed the most serious threat to the country. No other microbial agent was a contender. It was one of the most lethal of possible agents, killing 30% of its victims, and there was no available therapy.[1]

At the time, the US National Pharmaceutical Stockpile (later renamed the Strategic National Stockpile) held 15 million doses of smallpox vaccine, and official steps were taken quickly to acquire enough vaccine (over 300 million doses) for every US citizen to be vaccinated.[2] In 2002 the government started planning how to use the vaccines in preparation for a smallpox-based biological attack. A proposal for universal vaccination was rejected. In December the government instead announced an unprecedented mass campaign of smallpox vaccinations to be carried out in two phases: 500,000 military personnel and 500,000 health workers in phase one, and up to 10 million emergency response personnel (police, firefighters, etc.) in phase two.[3]

As a biosecurity practice the campaign promised a twofold public health benefit: vaccination would provide lasting protection (immunity) from infection to those individuals who would play critical response roles in the event of an attack involving *variola major*, and the chances of such an attack would be reduced if potential attackers calculated that the health damage caused would be less. The need for this benefit was neither clear nor present, however, and President George W. Bush described the vaccinations as "a precaution only and not a response to any information concerning imminent danger."[4] Certainly, the danger of *natural* exposure to the eradicated smallpox virus was nonexistent, yet real risks accompanied the process of vaccination. Principally, potential costs to would-be recipients of smallpox vaccine included its known side effects. Smallpox vaccination involves exposing individuals to a live virus (*vaccinia*) that is closely related to *variola major*. It comes with a high rate of complications ranging from scarring to death. Thus, in the absence of a risk of naturally occurring smallpox infection, and given the uncertainty about the risk of a biological attack, an individual could well perceive the risk of vaccination (complications) to outweigh the risk of remaining unvaccinated (vulnerability to a smallpox attack). Beyond personal health concerns, a large-scale smallpox vaccination campaign also generated another kind of problem: it partly interrupted the everyday activities of state and local health systems throughout the United States. As the campaign proceeded, some public health officials complained that, in order to meet its requirements, there had to be a scaling back of other important work such as TB screening and the administering of standard childhood inoculations.[5] It appeared to be an instance, then, of attention to smallpox (a nonexistent disease) occasioning neglect of ongoing health challenges. This concern about public health opportunity costs, combined with the concern about the potential personal costs, ultimately caused US health workers to overwhelmingly reject the option of undergoing smallpox vaccination. Less than eight percent of those targeted volunteered to participate in the Bush Administration's campaign. Seemingly very few had perceived that the biological attack risk outweighed the vaccination risk, and indeed the latter manifested in 145 cases of serious adverse reactions, including three that resulted in death.[6] Some supporters of the campaign criticized those who questioned or rejected it, arguing that the job of "physicians and hospital officials . . . is not to assess intelligence risks or second guess public health officials."[7] But that is exactly what most health workers did, and it happened because of a fundamental disharmony of emphasis between national security and public health.

In this example of biosecurity practice in the form of "civilian biodefense," real risks and measurable costs were seen as clearly outweighing an uncertain risk and potential (and unmeasurable) benefits. It is a lesson in the need for governments to consider carefully the benefits to be derived from a particular approach to the threat of biological attacks against the associated harms. In the United States this need persists in respect of other biosecurity practices aimed at protecting the general population and, as this chapter will show, the challenge that arises in this context is to achieve greater protection against biological attacks without thereby neglecting other serious health issues and health-protective measures. The challenge is an extremely difficult one for a government seeking to invest taxpayers' money wisely, largely because the setting of priorities and the allocating of resources cannot be based solely on accumulated evidence of the health burdens. That is, as a matter of biosecurity policy there is no way of reliably balancing the *known* burden of ongoing infectious disease risks against the *unknown* burden of future biological attacks. This means that the attention or neglect dilemma cannot be avoided simply by devoting a degree of attention to a given risk that evidence indicates is the "right" degree, even though this would seem to be the best way to maximize the public health utility of a biosecurity practice. Accordingly, the proposition to be explored is that spending on civilian biodefense should be guided by an ethic of "security-sensitive utilitarianism" and require that activities in this area yield a dual benefit (protection against both naturally occurring disease outbreaks and biological attacks). The chapter begins with an explanation of the foundations of this proposition, and this is followed by an assessment of two specific projects undertaken in the United States for civilian biodefense purposes: the disease surveillance project BioWatch and the drug development project BioShield.

DISEASE, UTILITY, AND SECURITY

Public health decision makers are traditionally attracted to policymaking that is based on assessment and analysis of consequences, both good and bad. This reflects a utilitarian ethic according to which the right choice (e.g., about how to allocate scarce resources) is the one that produces the most gain (e.g., the largest reduction in the burden of disease). When Jeremy Bentham (1748–1832) contemplated the consequences of decisions in terms of their impact on the well-being of affected individuals, he identified the moral imperative to achieve the greatest happiness of the greatest number.[8] Today it is possible to identify at least two kinds of utilitarians. Subjective utilitarians believe that well-being is best defined by each individual's personal experience; objective utilitarians prefer a centralized approach that involves experts defining an index of "rationally knowable" components of well-being.[9] Both focus on consequences and both are concerned to use resources in such a way as to generate the most good. But different conceptions of "the good" can lead to disagreements over policies and approaches preferred among subjective and objective utilitarians. For example, whereas many subjective utilitarians favor the use of markets to allocate healthcare resources (because markets respond to individual preferences), objective utilitarians tend to prefer "rational," data-driven processes of resource allocation.[10]

A heavy emphasis on individuals' subjective judgments could produce outcomes in policymaking that objective utilitarians would tend to regard as irrational. One example of this might be a degree of political concern about "new" risks that is greater than the concern about ongoing risks of similar magnitude. In the United States the risk posed by biological weapons is not new to a government that until 1969 maintained an offensive biological warfare program, but biological attacks could (beginning in late 2001) be plausibly characterized as a newly rediscovered risk. Subjective utilitarians—individually, and as a matter of individual preference—might overestimate such a risk and favor maximization of the "good" of personal security against biological attack. The US government, if responsive to a widespread expression of this preference, might in turn see political utility and value for (taxpayers') money by investing heavily in biodefense measures directed specifically against biological attacks. However, objective utilitarians would tend to argue that effort to reduce an overestimated risk is unjustified, and in so doing they would likely point to accumulated evidence of the burden of disease.

At the time of writing, the US government's list of biological "select agents" included thirteen Tier 1 agents (see Table 8.1) that are considered dangerous enough (for biological weapons purposes) to attract the most stringent laboratory biosecurity regulations. Only nine of the twelve diseases included on that list (botulism being mentioned twice) present a natural-occurrence risk to human

Table 8.1 Tier 1 Select Agents

Agent	Disease
botulinum neurotoxins	botulism
botulinum neurotoxin producing species of Clostridium	botulism
Ebola virus	Ebola
Francisella tularensis	tularemia
Marburg virus	Marburg hemorrhagic fever
Variola major	smallpox
Variola minor	alastrim
Yersinia pestis	plague
Bacillus anthracis	anthrax
Burkholderia mallei	glanders
Burkholderia pseudomallei	melioidosis
foot-and-mouth disease virus	foot-and-mouth disease
Rinderpest virus	rinderpest

Source: "Select Agents and Toxins List," Federal Select Agent Program 2014, http://www .selectagents.gov/SelectAgentsandToxinsList.html.

health because two of them do not affect humans (foot-and-mouth disease and rinderpest) and one was eradicated decades ago (smallpox). Of the nine remaining diseases caused by Tier 1 select agents, cases of only three—tularemia, botulism, and plague—were reported in the United States in 2013 (see Table 8.2).

On the basis of these figures and similar figures from previous years, it is reasonable to conclude that diseases caused by (Tier 1) pathogens of biological weapons concern are not a large ongoing problem in the United States.[11] Accordingly, the sizable amount of government funding devoted to resisting those diseases since 2001 has been the subject of complaint by analysts who adopt an objective utilitarian perspective (see chapter 2). In essence, their argument is that the US government gives too much attention to and spends too much money on civilian biodefense (or, at least, on the wrong kinds of biodefense), which results in too little effort and money being directed toward areas where more lives could be saved. For example, Hillel Cohen and his colleagues wrote in 2004 that "bioterrorism preparedness programs are . . . characterized by failure to apply reasonable priorities in the context of public health and failure to fully weigh the risks against the purported benefits of these programs."[12] The following year, Larry Gostin argued that "biodefense unfavorably shifts the public-health agenda to low-probability events, [and] funds the wrong activities."[13] A similar argument was advanced by 750 NIH-funded scientists in an open letter to the institutes' director. These

Table 8.2 Reported Cases of Selected Notifiable Diseases in the United States, 2013

Disease	Number of reported cases
chlamydia	1,401,906
gonorrhea	333,004
syphilis	56,471
salmonellosis	50,364
HIV infection	34,969
varicella (chickenpox)	11,359
tularemia*	203
botulism*	152
plague*	4
anthrax*	0
smallpox*	0

* Disease caused by a Tier 1 select agent (see Table 8.1).

Source: "Summary of Notifiable Infectious Diseases and Conditions—United States, 2013," *Morbidity and Mortality Weekly Report,* October 23, 2015, http://www.cdc.gov/mmwr/pre view/mmwrhtml/mm6253a1.htm.

scientists, observing the "massive influx of funding, institutions, and investigators into work on prioritized bioweapon agents," lamented the "diversion of research funds from projects of high public-health importance to projects of high biodefense but low public-health importance."[14] In 2007 Lynn Klotz claimed that "bioweapons agents are no natural public health threat" in the United States and argued that the "biggest need" was "an increase in funding for research and countermeasure development for endemic infectious diseases."[15] In 2010 the US-based Scientists Working Group on Biological and Chemical Weapons argued, "Continuing to emphasize and spend billions of dollars on measures to specifically counter exaggerated bioterrorist threats diverts attention and resources from other pressing natural disease threats and public health concerns."[16]

For at least three reasons, however, it is difficult to accept claims that the problem of biological attacks is afforded too much political attention based on health burden evidence alone. First, a flaw in the logic employed by objective utilitarians is the assumption that the risk of biological attacks is *necessarily* very low. Ironically, this flaw pertains to (lack of) evidence, and it is more accurate to regard that risk as being of an *uncertain* magnitude. The sparse empirical record of biological attacks in the United States and elsewhere could, on its own, support an argument that the US government's huge investment in measures for population defense is irrational and excessive only if that sparseness were certain to persist indefinitely. Added to this is the problem of assessing the risk of biological attacks *alongside* naturally occurring infectious disease risks, which arises from the fact that the latter have no element of agency. Disease resulting from malicious human action is distinguishable from a natural disease outbreak that will (as abundant experience shows) eventually run its course, which makes the health burden of biological attacks less amenable to prediction and management. Most important, an attacker who cannot be located and stopped *could* (but might not) strike again and keep striking. This critical element of uncertainty thus limits the value of an objective utilitarian approach to biodefense prioritization, so the attention or neglect dilemma is not avoided simply by recourse to accumulated data on past public health burdens.

A third reason why a government cannot straightforwardly devote greater attention to what evidence shows are the greater health burdens is that, in practice, policymakers (especially in a democracy) need to be responsive to public sentiment. In particular, government must be cognizant of and sensitive to people's desires not just to avoid death per se but also to avoid certain (dreaded) ways of dying. Although the WHO refers to mortality statistics all the time in describing the health burden of various diseases, it has acknowledged that individual deaths are qualitatively different from each other. For example, the 2002 World Health Report noted that using "number of deaths" as a measure "may not distinguish deaths of people who engage in an activity by choice and benefit from it directly, from those of people who are exposed to a hazard involuntarily and who get no direct benefits."[17] In the United States tens of thousands of people die each year on highways; on average scores of them do every day. However, as Lee Clarke has observed, this is generally not regarded as a "never-ending catastrophe" because, despite the prevalence of fatal car crashes, people "feel in control" of their vehicles and they benefit (e.g., financially) from driving regularly.[18] No such feeling accompanies the prospect of a deadly infection, though, for the experience of this hazard would be neither voluntary nor beneficial. Moreover, death resulting from an infectious disease can also sometimes be a fearsomely gruesome affair involving horrific symptoms such as disfiguring skin eruptions (anthrax) or massive hemorrhaging (Ebola). Whereas it is frightening enough to contemplate the natural occurrence of these and other dreaded diseases, more fear is probably inspired by the notion of being subjected to maliciously deliberate infection.

A state of affairs in which statistics are subordinated to emotion is anathema to an objective utilitarian. Nevertheless, in the context of popular dread of biological attacks, the feasibility of priority-setting that is strictly based on previous evidence is liable to be undermined by a widespread attitude that "the possibilities are more worrisome than the probabilities."[19] It seems unreasonable, then, to expect that a government could simply be "beaten over the head" with evidence and bludgeoned into prioritizing resources "rationally." Although a concern to maximize the public health utility of civilian biodefense as a biosecurity practice remains valid, it would arguably be more useful to temper that concern with sensitivity to people's desire for security against dreaded risks of uncertain magnitude. Given that in matters of public health and national security governments must contemplate and address not just what is happening but also what might happen in the future, a better form of utilitarianism to guide biodefense priority-setting is one that is "security sensitive." Such an ethic would constitute a *via media* between objective utilitarianism that is dispassionately evidence-based on the one hand and subjective utilitarianism driven by people's dread of being attacked on the other. The compromise approach would be to require all civilian biodefense projects to afford protection against natural as well as intentional infectious disease risks; biosecurity practice in this area would need to satisfy a dual-benefit test of its utility.

DUAL-BENEFIT BIODEFENSE

The fulfilment of a dual-benefit requirement would not perfectly surmount the attention or neglect dilemma that potentially arises from civilian biodefense activities in the United States. However, it could go some way to assuaging concerns that the US biodefense boom detrimentally draws attention and resources away from important areas of public health activity in the way that the 2003 smallpox vaccination campaign attempted to do. When the boom began, the large increase in government funding for biological attack preparedness was generally regarded as good news from a public health perspective. For example, an editorial in *The Lancet* stated:

> Some of the money being appropriated for biological defence in the USA will go into improved disease surveillance and outbreak detection, and upgrading of a public-health system that has been under-funded for too long. . . . The long-term spin-off benefit for infectious disease surveillance as a whole is to be welcomed . . . although the money being spent to protect against bioterrorism is probably not proportional to the immediate risk, an improvement in public protection against all transmissible diseases is likely.[20]

Two years later, though, four US health officials warned, "If our public health planning efforts are too narrowly focused on preparing responses to a few select bioterrorism-related scenarios, a new opportunity for planning responses to a broad spectrum of infectious disease-related catastrophes will be lost."[21] Such a prospect indeed seemed likely during the presidency of George W. Bush, when the US federal government warned state health authorities "not to use bioter-rorism funds for general [public health] purposes."²² Under President Barack Obama, however, the emphasis changed. According to Gregory Koblentz, there was a shift in thinking away from Bush's concept of "biodefence (measures to pre-pare for and respond to the intentional use of disease as a weapon)" and toward Obama's concept of "biosecurity (measures to prevent, prepare for and respond to both naturally occurring and deliberately engineered biological threats)."²³ That shift has been reflected in federal budget figures, which, at the time of writ-ing, evidenced a continuing decrease in emphasis on measures aimed *solely* at protecting the US population against biological attacks.²⁴ Increasingly, then, US government-funded measures for responding to and mitigating attacks are in some way beneficial *also* when it comes to infectious disease risks more generally. Nevertheless, it remains the case that some ongoing civilian biodefense projects do not fare well when the dual-benefit test for utility is applied. Two such projects worthy of particular attention are BioWatch and BioShield.

The BioWatch Project and Disease Surveillance

BioWatch is a surveillance system intended to achieve protection only against biological attacks through the early detection of pathogenic microorganisms deliberately disseminated into the air. As such, the project immediately fails the dual-benefit test. Even so, some discussion of the operation of this system as a biosecurity practice is worthwhile because it illustrates the claim that US gov-ernment spending on biodefense is sometimes ill-directed. BioWatch consists of placing environmental sensors throughout thirty US cities and at major spectator events that automatically sample the surrounding air several times a day. Vacuum pumps draw the air through filters that catch airborne microorganisms; the filters are retrieved daily and taken to public health laboratories, where they are tested for the presence of pathogens named on a list maintained by the DHS. The list is secret, but in 2009 a DHS official told *USA Today*: "We're looking for aerosol-ized anthrax [bacteria]. That's the No. 1 aerosolized biological risk agent."²⁵ The names of the cities in which BioWatch operates are secret, too, but the system has reportedly triggered alarms in Los Angeles, Detroit, St. Louis, Phoenix, San Diego, and San Francisco.²⁶ As time (for response) is of the essence in the event of a biological attack, one supposed benefit of the BioWatch system is that it can detect an attack earlier than ordinary disease-surveillance systems would. The US government then would be alerted to the occurrence of a biological attack at or shortly after the moment when a pathogen was released into the air rather than days or weeks later when exposure to that pathogen started causing disease in human victims. Another benefit, attributable in part to the secrecy surrounding the pathogens being monitored and the location of BioWatch sensors, is deterrence. The idea is that, if would-be users of biological weapons suspect that an attack using any pathogen could be detected anywhere and anytime, they are less likely to bother with an attack that would cause little or no damage thanks to the local health system's rapid response to a detection alarm.

The pursuit of these benefits has come at a high financial cost: the US government allocated $876 million in total to BioWatch during the period FY2007 through FY2016.[27] However, the protective value of the system as a whole is reduced by the frequency with which it has generated false alarms. Ned Calonge, chief medical officer of the Colorado Department of Public Health and Environment from 2002 to 2010, told the *Los Angeles Times* in 2012: "The only times it goes off, it's wrong. I just think it's a colossal waste of money. It's a stupid program."[28] The essential problem is that BioWatch sensors are oversensitive to microorganisms other than those that the system is intended to detect. Closely related but nonpathogenic organisms that exist naturally in the environment are mistaken for pathogenic organisms that are present as the result of deliberate dissemination. The frequency of false alarms has led local health officials to reportedly lose confidence in BioWatch.[29] Thus, in practice the system cannot be counted on to detect *and* set in motion a response to a real biological attack. Moreover, some of the US government's own scientists reportedly think that BioWatch probably cannot protect against the most likely form of a biological attack (small-scale releases of pathogens) and that the system would struggle to detect even a large-scale release.[30] In both instances the difficulty would be that disease-causing microorganisms present in the air surrounding a sensor could be at concentrations too low to trigger a BioWatch alarm.

Despite the problems of pathogen-detection technology, BioWatch still attracts some support on national security grounds. For example, Steven Bucci from the Heritage Foundation argued:

> BioWatch isn't perfect. But it's a huge improvement over what we had before, which was nothing . . . yes, BioWatch is very costly. But the dangers it aims to mitigate are catastrophic. What leader is prepared to stand before the American people and say, "Well, we might have been able to detect that bio-weapon before it killed thousands of innocents, but BioWatch might not have saved everyone . . . and just think of all the money we saved by pulling the plug!" . . . Just because a system is not perfect does not mean it is not valuable, or that it does not protect American lives.[31]

When contemplating the utility of a biosecurity practice, however, it is arguably not enough to be satisfied that that practice achieves *some* benefit at *any* cost. Rather, what matters is the balance of benefits and costs, including opportunity costs. In the case of BioWatch, the problem is not just that its dubious benefits—detection and deterrence—are expensive but also that the system consumes attention and resources that might otherwise be fruitfully directed toward other disease-surveillance activities. As such, it could be regarded as worse than (not an improvement on) "nothing."[32] A better biosecurity practice would be to invest in disease surveillance measures that *can* detect the occurrence of a biological attack (albeit not instantly); the additional benefit likely to be derived from this would be an improved capacity to detect naturally occurring outbreaks too. A dual benefit could be achieved, for example, by upgrading bioinformatics systems that pick up unusual disease patterns and by improving diagnostic capabilities at hospitals that receive people presenting with symptoms of infectious disease. Yet, while the BioWatch system continues to attract attention and resources, a degree of opportunity to pursue these other activities is lost.

Project BioShield and Pharmaceutical Countermeasures

There is an opportunity cost associated with BioShield, too, although this civilian biodefense project has the potential to afford a dual benefit. Project BioShield is a multibillion-dollar incentive scheme that encourages pharmaceutical companies to conduct research on pathogens of biological weapons concern. The research is conducted with a view to developing and producing large quantities of new and better drugs (vaccines, antibiotics, antitoxins, and antiviral drugs), which are then sold to the US government, which in turn stores and replenishes the drugs in the Strategic National Stockpile (SNS) to be used in a public health emergency such as a biological attack. When President Bush proposed BioShield in his 2003 State of the Union speech, he predicted that this "major research and production effort to guard our people against bioterrorism" would "quickly make available effective vaccines and treatments against agents like anthrax, botulinum toxin, Ebola, and plague."[33] The following year, Congress approved funding of $5.6 billion over the ten years to 2014. Accompanying legislation enabled the hiring of personnel and the securing of facilities for BioShield-funded research to be expedited, and it also allowed the FDA to make experimental (i.e., not fully tested) drugs available in emergencies.[34]

As a biosecurity practice, the expending of effort and resources through Project BioShield promises two benefits. The first is that the large quantity of drugs delivered to the SNS could be used to prevent widespread illness and death in the event of a biological attack involving a pathogen against which a stockpiled drug is effective. This is particularly appealing from a disease-control perspective because the availability of pharmaceutical resources to defeat a *contagious* disease would reduce the need to implement disruptive nonpharmaceutical measures of the kind discussed in Part III (like border control and quarantine). The second benefit—deterrence—is based on a supposition that the likelihood of an attack being attempted is lower if a potential attacker thinks the adverse health effects would be limited by the availability of prophylactic or therapeutic drugs. In an attempt to deny attackers the option of using anthrax bacteria, for example, the US government adopts a three-pronged approach.[35] In addition to vaccines and antibiotics, the third "prong" is anthrax antitoxin usable against antibiotic-resistant strains of *Bacillus anthracis*. According to former US Navy secretary Richard Danzig, the benefit of this approach is that it "complicate[s] an attacker's strategy, just as the bomber-land-missile-submarine triad complicates a would-be nuclear attacker's task."[36]

A number of factors can potentially diminish the expected benefit of BioShield. One of these is the fact that the program has produced, and currently aims only to produce, pharmaceutical countermeasures against an extremely narrow range of pathogenic microorganisms. Since the disbursement of BioShield grants began in 2005, not every grant has resulted in a usable new drug and, according to a 2015 report by the DHHS, BioShield acquisitions are usable against only three diseases: anthrax, botulism, and smallpox (see Table 8.3). A determined attacker could instead set out to cause a disease against which a drug is not available (i.e., held in the SNS) or stage an attack using a pathogen genetically engineered to resist existing vaccines or treatments. In addition, a question arising from the newness of the drugs developed and stockpiled through BioShield is, Will they actually work in the event of an attack? Tests of the new smallpox vaccine Imvamune˚ have shown that it is safe and well-tolerated by recipients, but there has been no opportunity to test this vaccine's effectiveness against actual smallpox infection. Because the anthrax antitoxin Raxibacumab,˚ which was licensed for emergency use in December 2012 under the FDA's Animal Efficacy Rule, has not been shown to work against anthrax infection in humans, there is a chance it might turn out to be useless in the event of a biological attack.[37] Lastly, the benefit afforded by drugs procured through BioShield might in practice be available to too few people, especially in the event that an attacker used a human-to-human transmissible microorganism to spark contagion. Even if infections resulting from a biological attack were susceptible to existing treatments, and assuming that stockpiled drugs could be distributed quickly, the number of individual illnesses caused might be so great as to exceed the lifesaving capacity of the SNS.

Table 8.3 Select BioShield Pharmaceutical Countermeasure Acquisitions by the End of 2012

Countermeasure	Stockpile status	Total funding
anthrax therapeutics		
Raxibacumab® (antitoxin)	65,000 doses delivered	$334 million
Anthrax Immune Globulin (antitoxin)	10,000 doses delivered	$160.6 million
anthrax vaccines		
BioThrax®	28.75 million doses delivered	$699.7 million
Recombinant Protective Antigen	(contract terminated in 2005)	$2 million
botulism therapeutics		
botulinum antitoxin (hBAT) Therapeutic	148,702 doses and plasma delivered (of 200,000 contracted)	$476 million
smallpox vaccines		
Imvamune®	28 million doses delivered (of 28 million contracted)	$770 million
smallpox antivirals		
ST-246 (Arestvyr)	1.2 million treatment courses delivered (of 1.7 million contracted)	$433 million

Source: "Project BioShield Annual Report to Congress, January 2014–December 2014," US Department of Health and Human Services, 2015, https://www.medicalcountermeasures.gov/media/36816/pbs-report-2014.pdf, 6–8.

If indeed BioShield is not sufficiently protective of the US population, some might believe that the US government has thus far invested too little effort and resources in an otherwise worthwhile biodefense activity. In the absence of government intervention it is almost certain that market forces alone would not have brought about the development and production of drugs like Imvamune® and Raxibacumab®. Nevertheless, experience has shown that BioShield's original $5.6 billion—a "spit in the bucket," according to Robert Kadlec—has not been enough to attract the interest of large and experienced pharmaceutical companies with well-established R&D programs.[38] It seems unlikely that such companies will be attracted to the additional $2.8 billion that Congress has made available over the five years to 2018. However, even if these amounts were higher, a fundamental problem would remain: the commercial incentive to treat ongoing health risks is far greater than the incentive to help a single customer (i.e., the US government) resist the uncertain risk of attacks that cause otherwise rare diseases. If BioShield were directed toward a broader range of infectious disease risks, and if the drugs produced could be used regularly as well as stockpiled, the commercial incentive to engage with the project would probably be greater. Moreover, because a project of this kind would better satisfy the dual-benefit test, it would have greater utility as a biosecurity practice.

If, according to an ethic of security-sensitive utilitarianism, a biosecurity practice is required to afford a dual benefit, the most conspicuous failing of BioShield is its purchase of $1.6 billion worth of new drugs to defeat smallpox, a disease that no longer exists. These drugs offer only a single benefit: protection against the nonnatural emergence of *variola major*. The enormous cost, difficult to justify on public health grounds, precludes expenditure on pharmaceutical-based biosecurity practices that would likely be more beneficial over time. The cost of procuring the antiviral drug Arestvyr™, for example, has been around $200 per dose, and a justification for this by reference only to the risk of a biological attack has apparently been insufficient to sway opinion. Rather, the drug's proponents have sought also to justify the high cost by reference to health risks that (unlike smallpox) are ongoing. Robin Robinson, director of the federal government's Biomedical Advanced Research and Development Authority, has described $200 as a "fair and reasonable" price, given that other antiviral drugs sell for between $108 and $7,364. Eric Rose, president of Siga Technologies (which manufactures Arestvyr™), has claimed it is "a bargain" compared to the annual cost of $20,000 for AIDS antiretrovirals and cancer drugs that cost more than $100,000. Moreover, Rose has reasoned that the US government's order for fewer than 2 million doses is "on the low end," given that "there are 80 million doses of Tamiflu in the strategic national stockpile" and that "smallpox is just as contagious [as influenza] and has thirty times the mortality."[39] What these justifications ignore, however, is that the *natural* occurrence of smallpox is impossible (in stark contrast to influenza, AIDS, and cancer). It was probably for this very reason that in 2003 so many health workers refused to participate in the government's smallpox vaccination campaign.

A good starting point, then, in converting BioShield into a more cost-effective, dual-benefit biosecurity enterprise would be either to abandon the pursuit of new smallpox-defeating drugs or to pursue these only if they are protective also against disease outbreaks that occur naturally. The latter option would move BioShield away from a targeted "one bug, one drug" approach to drug development and toward the pursuit of "broad-spectrum" pharmaceutical countermeasures usable against a variety of infections. Such drugs, which are presently hypothetical, would be of greater utility for ongoing public health purposes and would also afford better protection against biological attacks (including, perhaps, those involving genetically engineered pathogens). However, drugs of this kind are more likely to come about as a result of research inquiring at a fundamental level into the behavior of microorganisms and pathogen-host interaction. The research currently encouraged by BioShield tends to be "applied" rather than "basic," and although it has the potential to yield scientific discoveries of a fundamental nature, the relative difficulty of working with a pathogen of biological weapons concern (*Bacillus anthracis*, for example) lessens that potential. Microbiologists in general are less familiar with anthrax bacteria than they are with standard-model bacteria like *Escherichia coli*, so the advantage of studying the latter in a laboratory is that it can be done without the need for stringent biosafety and biosecurity measures to be in place.

Basic research with a view to developing broad-spectrum pharmaceuticals would be a longer-term element of a dual-benefit BioShield, while in the meantime an element of targeted research for drug development purposes could afford protection against both intentional and nonintentional infectious disease risks. Already, new drugs have been acquired to treat anthrax and botulism, which, in addition to being diseases of biological weapons concern, are a natural but low-level burden to US public health (see Table 8.2). It may be, though, that the volume of anti-anthrax and anti-botulism drugs acquired through BioShield is excessive, given that neither disease is contagious. Rather than maintaining, for example, enough anthrax vaccine to respond to a "three-city attack," arguably it would be sufficient to maintain a much smaller supply in readiness for the occasional naturally occurring case of anthrax or for an anthrax attack that is more likely to occur on a small scale than on a large one.[40] This would reduce the ongoing expense of the stockpile since each year the US government reportedly disposes of expired doses of anthrax vaccine worth around $48 million.[41] It also would free up resources for addressing the greater risk posed by dreaded diseases that are human-to-human transmissible. Prioritizing the acquisition of new drugs to defeat the Ebola virus, for example, would be beneficial in respect of a future Ebola-based biological attack in the United States. Even if such an attack never occurred, the availability of vaccines or antivirals would afford a valuable alternative to the nonpharmaceutical biosecurity practices that proved so troublesome during the 2014 Ebola outbreak in West Africa.

CONCLUSION

In December 2002, after President Bush announced his smallpox vaccination campaign, a US health official offered the justification "Given the world situation, the uncertainty of the threat, the number of voices and noises out there, and the combination of public health and political considerations, this isn't a bad place to be."[42] This official utterance, far from being evidence-based, reflected a situation in which an urgent concern for national security had overwhelmed the usual tendency of public health practitioners toward objective utilitarianism. Where was the *evidence* of a real health burden, they might have asked, on which a decision to prioritize effort and resources in this way could be based? Then, as now, vaccination against smallpox made sense only by reference to the uncertain risk of a biological attack using *variola major* because the disease that virus causes was nowhere in existence. When Bush's vaccination campaign eventually failed as a biosecurity practice, it was because so many of those to be immunized regarded this as the assumption more than the avoidance of a personal risk and because the campaign consumed attention in a way that occasioned neglect of ongoing health problems.

In the period since, the potential for the US government again to fall foul of the attention or neglect dilemma has persisted, and it has frequently been accused of affording an unjustifiably high degree of attention to the risk of future biological attacks. However, it would be a mistake for critics (objective utilitarians) simply to dismiss such emphasis as irrational and to demand that the prioritization of effort and expenditure be entirely evidence-based. Such a demand, though intended to encourage maximization of human well-being, is one that disregards the responsibility of governments to accommodate uncertainty about the future and to be sensitive to the fears of its citizens. In the face of a strong, popular desire to be protected against the possibility of deliberate infection with a dreaded disease, a better approach would be to allow efforts toward that end to proceed and to demand that such efforts be protective also against infectious disease risks of natural origin. In this way concerns about the public health utility of civilian biodefense activities would be addressed at least partly and governments would retain a degree of political flexibility in undertaking this form of biosecurity practice.

In the United States most government-funded activity in the area of civilian biodefense is already of a kind that promises or achieves a dual benefit. However, as this discussion has shown, the utility of some activities remains open to question. In the case of BioWatch, the problem begins with the fact that the system struggles in practice to produce its intended single benefit: reliable early warning of a biological attack. In addition, the technical features of BioWatch are such that it is a bad system in principle, casting its one-eyed gaze on the problem of biological weapons only. BioWatch contributes nothing to the surveillance of infectious disease risks more generally, and the high financial cost of maintaining the system draws effort and resources away from dual-benefit disease-surveillance activities that are effective even if able to be improved. The drug-procurement project BioShield, by contrast, is in principle a good idea with plenty of dual-benefit potential. New drugs to defeat dreaded diseases are less likely to be produced by pharmaceutical companies in the absence of a financial incentive, and it is generally preferable for a government to be able to use drug supplies (rather than social distancing) to control an outbreak of natural or deliberate origin. Even so, there is scope for BioShield to perform better as a biosecurity practice. The pursuit of new smallpox drugs (which promises only the single benefit of protection against a nonnatural outbreak) could be abandoned, and drugs for defeating noncontagious diseases could be stockpiled in much smaller amounts. Thereafter, a greater degree of attention could be directed toward contagious diseases with transnational reach and toward the encouragement of research into broad-spectrum drugs.

NOTES

1. D. A. Henderson, "Smallpox Epidemic Models and Response Strategies," *Biosecurity and Bioterrorism* 11, no. 1 (2013): 74.
2. Wil S. Hylton, "How Ready Are We for Bioterrorism?," *New York Times*, October 30, 2011, MM26.
3. Hillel W. Cohen, Robert M. Gould, and Victor W. Sidel, "The Pitfalls of Bioterrorism Preparedness: The Anthrax and Smallpox Experiences," *American Journal of Public Health* 94, no. 10 (2004): 1668.
4. Matthew Benns, "Smallpox Vaccine," *Sun Herald* (Sydney), December 15, 2002, 10.
5. Cohen, Gould, and Sidel, "Pitfalls," 1669. See also Institute of Medicine, *The Smallpox Vaccination Program: Public Health in an Age of Terrorism* (Washington, DC: National Academies Press, 2005).
6. Debora Mackenzie, "US Smallpox Vaccination Plan Grinds to a Halt," *New Scientist*, August 22, 2003, www.newscientist.com/article/dn4074-us-smallpox-vaccination-plan-grinds-to-a-halt.html.
7. Ceci Connolly, "Two Large Hospitals Refuse Smallpox Shots," *Washington Post*, December 18, 2002, A02.
8. See Jeremy Bentham, *The Principles of Morals and Legislation* (Oxford: Clarendon, 1996 [1789]).
9. Marc J. Roberts and Michael R. Reich, "Ethical Analysis in Public Health," *The Lancet* 359 (March 23, 2002): 1055.
10. Ibid., 1055–56.
11. See Centers for Disease Control and Prevention, *"Morbidity and Mortality Weekly Report*: Summary of Notifiable Infectious Diseases," October 22, 2015, http://www.cdc.gov/mmwr/mmwr_nd/.
12. Cohen, Gould, and Sidel, "Pitfalls," 1667.
13. Lawrence O. Gostin, "Finding a Space for the Public's Health in Bioterrorism Funding: A Commentary," *American Journal of Bioethics* 5, no. 4 (2005): 46.
14. Sidney Altman et al., "An Open Letter to Elias Zerhouni," *Science* 307, no. 5714 (2005): 1409.

15. Lynn Klotz, "Casting a Wider Net for Countermeasure R&D Funding Decision," *Biosecurity and Bioterrorism* 5, no. 4 (2007): 317.

16. Scientists Working Group on Biological and Chemical Weapons, "Biological Threats: A Matter of Balance," *Bulletin of the Atomic Scientists*, February 2, 2010, http://thebulletin.org/biological-threats-matter-balance.

17. World Health Organization, *Reducing Risks, Promoting Healthy Life* (World Health Report 2002) (2002), 34.

18. Lee Clarke, *Worst Cases: Terror and Catastrophe in the Popular Imagination* (Chicago: University of Chicago Press, 2006), 12.

19. Ibid., 78.

20. Editorial, "What Good Can Come of This?," *The Lancet Infectious Diseases* 1, no. 11 (2001): 213.

21. Kathleen F. Gensheimer, Martin I. Meltzer, Alicia S. Postema, and Raymond A. Strikas, "Influenza Pandemic Preparedness," *Emerging Infectious Diseases* 9, no. 12 (2003): 1647.

22. Gostin, "Finding a Space," 46.

23. Gregory D. Koblentz, "From Biodefence to Biosecurity: The Obama Administration's Strategy for Countering Biological Threats," *International Affairs* 88, no. 1 (2012): 132.

24. See Tara Kirk Sell and Matthew Watson, "Federal Agency Biodefense Funding, FY2013–FY2014," *Biosecurity and Bioterrorism* 11, no. 3 (2013): 196–216; and Crystal Boddie, Tara Kirk Sell, and Matthew Watson, "Federal Funding for Health Security in FY2016," *Health Security* 13, no. 3 (2015): 186–206.

25. Steve Sternberg, "Behind the Scenes, System Sniffs for Biological Attacks," *USA Today*, October 7, 2009, http://usatoday30.usatoday.com/news/health/2009-10-05-biowatch-biological_N.htm.

26. David Willman, "The Biodefender that Cries Wolf," *Los Angeles Times*, July 8, 2012, http://www.latimes.com/news/nationworld/nation/la-na-biowatch-20120708,0,5093512.story.

27. See Sell and Watson, "Federal Agency Biodefense Funding," 201; and Boddie, Sell, and Watson, "Federal Funding for Health Security in FY2016," 189.

28. Willman, "Biodefender that Cries Wolf."

29. Ibid.

30. David Willman, "BioWatch's Chief Aim Is Off-Target, U.S. Security Officials Say," *Los Angeles Times*, June 18, 2013, http://articles.latimes.com/2013/jun/18/nation/la-na-biowatch-20130619; Willman, "Biodefender that Cries Wolf."

31. Steven P. Bucci, "Bag BioWatch Because of Its Bugs? Bad Idea," *Los Angeles Times*, December 7, 2012, http://articles.latimes.com/2012/dec/07/news/la-ol-biowatch-blowback-20121207.

32. See ibid.

33. Jon Cohen, "Reinventing Project BioShield," *Science* 333 (September 2, 2011): 1216.

34. Mary Quirk, "Boost to U.S. National Security with Signing of BioShield," *The Lancet Infectious Diseases* 4, no. 9 (2004): 540.

35. US Department of Health and Human Services, "Project BioShield Annual Report to Congress, January 2012–December 2012," 2013, https://www.medicalcounter measures.gov/media/33065/pbs_report_2012_hires_final2_508.pdf, 6.

36. Richard Danzig, *Catastrophic Bioterrorism—What Is to Be Done?* (Washington, DC: National Defense University, 2003), 10.
37. Us Department of Health and Human Services, "Project BioShield Annual Report," 4.
38. J. Cohen, "Reinventing Project BioShield," 1217.
39. Donald G. McNeil, "U.S. Buys Smallpox Drug, but Some Question Cost," *New York Times*, March 13, 2013, A3.
40. Hylton, "How Ready Are We," MM26.
41. David Perera, "Up to $48M of Expired Anthrax Vaccine Thrown Out Annually, Says DHS Official," *Fierce Homeland Security*, April 18, 2012, http://www.fiercehomelandsecurity.com/story/48m-expired-anthrax-vaccine-thrown-out-annually-says-dhs-official/2012-04-18.
42. Jon Cohen and Martin Enserink, "Rough-and-Tumble behind Bush's Smallpox Policy," *Science* 298 (December 20, 2002): 2316.

CONCLUSION

SINCE 2011 THE CDC HAS ENGAGED in an online Zombie Preparedness campaign to encourage preparedness for public health emergencies. Products available on the campaign's website include free posters depicting a zombie, a "graphic novella which uses the idea of a zombie apocalypse to demonstrate the importance of preparedness," and a "zombie blog."[1] Ali Khan, as director of the CDC's Office of Public Health Preparedness and Response, has blogged that reading the centers' advice on what to do during a zombie apocalypse could enable people to "learn a thing or two about how to prepare for a *real* emergency" (emphasis in original).[2] He has offered readers the assurance

> Never fear . . . if zombies did start roaming the streets, CDC would conduct an investigation much like any other disease outbreak. CDC would provide technical assistance to cities, states, or international partners dealing with a zombie infestation. This assistance might include consultation, lab testing and analysis, patient management and care, tracking of contacts, and infection control (including isolation and quarantine).[3]

The campaign is obviously intended as a fun way to draw attention to public health emergencies that might actually happen, and yet it also reinforces the notion that some infectious diseases are to be dreaded. Zombieism, if it existed, would surely be the most fearsome disease of all. Although there are variations in the way zombie plagues are portrayed by novelists and filmmakers, the general idea is that an infection of this kind is incurable and unsurvivable. One hundred percent of people bitten by zombies are quickly turned into zombies themselves, and victims in a state of animated "undeath" are then driven to infect the living.[4] As a scenario of contagion it is both terrifying and fascinating, which explains the popularity of the zombie genre in film and literature. It is fortunate that no real disease outbreak would ever resemble it.

In real-world circumstances, though, there are still some infectious diseases that inspire enough dread and government concern as to be accorded the status of being security issues. Beyond the influence of popular culture, this special status could be due to a disease's historical reputation, the gruesome symptoms it causes, the unavailability of effective treatment, and the past or possible causation of a disease through a biological attack. Invoking "security" in the context of a dreaded disease is not always advantageous, however, notwithstanding the extra resources and extraordinary power for risk reduction that this commonly entails. Rather, as this book has shown, security-oriented efforts to prevent or respond to disease outbreaks (whether naturally occurring or arising from human action) have the potential to generate harms as well as benefits. In a variety of ways, biosecurity practices generate or exacerbate tensions between different interests and values and make it difficult for governments to decide how to go about protecting populations within and among states. In confronting these biosecurity dilemmas, the challenge is to somehow avoid such practices that tend to undermine rather than promote public health over time.

First, there is the protect or proliferate dilemma, which potentially arises from state-based efforts to defend against biological attacks. At the international level, in respect of some biodefense activities undertaken by governments for "threat assessment" purposes, the essential problem is one of offense-defense differentiation. That is, one state's activities, purportedly aimed at affording protection against pathogenic microorganisms that are deliberately disseminated, might be perceived by the government of another state as having an offensive purpose. If this suspicion occasions similar activities to occur in that other state (e.g., investigations into offensive capabilities), the result could be a proliferation of biological weapons risks and an increased likelihood of attacks while each side continues to compete for advantage. A protect or proliferate dilemma also can arise at the domestic level, although here the concern is a possible increase in the risk of an attack originating from within a state's biodefense enterprise. Where that enterprise is large scale, as it is in the United States, there is greater defensive potential, but there is also a greater probability of disease outbreaks resulting from a pathogen being stolen and maliciously misused by someone on the inside. The solution to this problem would appear to be a higher degree of regulation of scientific activities. But this in turn has the potential to generate a different, secure or stifle biosecurity dilemma. In moving to make research on pathogenic microorganisms more secure against accidents, theft, and the misuse of data, a government might end up stifling researchers' pursuit of discoveries that could one day lead to the saving of lives in the event of an outbreak. Although imposing and tightening regulations that govern laboratory work and technology transfers (both tangible and intangible) is protective in an immediate sense, over time it could become antiprotective if it adversely affected too many scientists' ability and willingness to investigate defenses against infectious disease risks. The conundrum, then, is that the securing of populations against dreaded diseases can seem at once to require both the restricting and the facilitating of research efforts.

A government's promotion of pathogen research, whether regulated to a greater or lesser degree, is driven mainly by a desire to develop drugs that prevent or cure disease. It is an important objective because, to the extent that such drugs are available, there is less need to protect population health by resorting to nonpharmaceutical disease-control measures. Drug development is a lengthy process, though, and in many countries a pharmaceutical response to a dreaded disease might not be available when it is needed. This could be due, for example, to vaccine-supply problems (as occurred with pandemic influenza) or a pathogen's resistance to existing antibiotics (such as with *Mycobacterium tuberculosis*). In these cases, once a feared disease outbreak is actually under way, a third kind of biosecurity dilemma might arise: remedy or overkill. When a government moves to frame an outbreak as a matter of national security, thus claiming a need to respond swiftly and aggressively, the benefit could be the obtaining of resources and powers that are necessary to contain contagion. However, the risk is that such a response might transgress normal rules and expectations in a way that is unjust and counterproductive to public health. In particular, infringements on people's freedom of movement within and between national territories could in some circumstances amount to the negative securitization of a disease. In a highly interconnected world, where microorganisms are as mobile as their human hosts, the policing of borders to prevent microbial incursion is often futile and thus an unnecessary interference with international traffic. A more promising alternative is for governments to pursue biosecurity in a cooperative fashion for the sake of populations that are collectively vulnerable to dreaded diseases with transnational reach. Here, too, another biosecurity dilemma can arise: attention or neglect. In the pursuit of an agenda of global health security as an international health governance arrangement, the challenge is to achieve extra protection against prioritized disease risks (including biological attacks) without simultaneously neglecting other health issues and national health-system weaknesses over the long term. Moreover, the setting of biosecurity policy priorities at the national level can present the same sort of challenge. Recent experience in the United States is instructive of the need for governments to consider carefully the benefits and harms associated with activities designed especially to protect a civilian population against biological attack. Whereas some such activities risk public health by soaking up scarce resources, others risk international proliferation of biological weapons. Thus the sequence of overlapping biosecurity dilemmas comes full circle.

Dilemmas are by nature resistant to straightforward solutions. As populations and governments continue to confront dreaded diseases, the imperatives of public health, national security, human rights, and scientific progress are likely to remain difficult generally to reconcile. However, in the course of this book's exploration of biosecurity dilemmas, a number of specific policies have been suggested as having the potential at least to reduce the tension between different interests and values.

First, regarding the protect or proliferate dilemma, a source of international proliferation pressure could be extinguished if the US government conspicuously abandoned and eschewed biodefense activities that are most liable to be perceived as having an offensive purpose. For example, as suggested in chapter 1, outdoor experimentation involving mechanisms for dispersing microorganisms on a large scale should be stopped on the grounds that such activity brings the "biological" far too close to the "weapon." In the absence of an international legal instrument for verifying a state's compliance with the BWC, external suspicion that a biological weapons threat exists is harder to dispel, and the risk is that some states might seek to keep pace with US microbe-dispersal capabilities. Experimentation with offensive capabilities so as to determine defensive requirements is probably more trouble than it is worth.

Second, with regard to the secure or stifle dilemma, the tension between the rival imperatives of restrictiveness and permissiveness in laboratory-based pathogen research could be lessened if researchers collectively embraced self-governance through codes of conduct. As discussed in chapter 3, to be reliant solely on regulations imposed from above is inadequate for the purpose of preventing attacks by scientist-bioterrorists, and very strict regulations might be an undue hindrance to beneficial scientific progress. Whereas the law is incapable of anticipating every security risk that might arise in a laboratory, a commitment to nonlegally binding codes of conduct could be more effective as a governance measure. Such codes could empower pathogen researchers in government, university, and commercial laboratories in order to preserve public trust in the work that they do and to champion its worth in public health terms. As a matter of professional responsibility, code-bound researchers would be required to weigh carefully the risks and benefits of their (intended) work in a timely, ongoing, consultative, and systematic fashion. In practice, commitment to a code of conduct could dispose a pathogen researcher to avoid risky activities voluntarily. Or, after following a rigorous weighing of risks and benefits, he or she could conscientiously press on in pursuit of a lifesaving discovery. Beyond that, researchers could also commit to going along with the policy suggested in chapter 4: "discreet dissemination" of any research findings that present too great a proliferation risk if conventionally published. As an alternative to censorship, this restrictive approach would still be permissive enough to address any public health need for data transfer and would serve as a reminder to ambitious researchers that accumulating notoriety within prestigious publications is not all that matters in their work.

Third, with regard to the remedy or overkill dilemma, the specific suggestion offered in chapter 5—that XDR-TB patients should be isolated in sanatoria—would be justified only if it amounted to the positive securitization of a dreaded disease. That is, the circumstances of isolation, as an extreme form of social distancing, would need to be such that it is effective but not counterproductive as a disease-control measure. Drug-resistant TB is a strong candidate for securitization by concerned governments, given that it is contagious and deadly while also being difficult and expensive to treat. If securitization occurs, though, the extraordinariness of the response that is warranted by the disease's security status should be such as would encourage victims to separate themselves from the general population voluntarily and indefinitely. In a sanatorium, unlike a prison, XDR-TB patients would need to enjoy as many economic and recreational opportunities as could reasonably be afforded to them. They should also be entitled to receive the best treatment available and to know that, beyond the sanatorium, a serious effort to prevent drug-resistant TB bacteria from emerging in the first place was under way.

Lastly, with regard to the attention or neglect dilemma, there is a case for requiring all civilian biodefense activities to be protective against natural disease outbreaks as well as biological attacks. As suggested in chapter 8, this dual-benefit requirement would be a compromise in the face of rival concerns that biological weapons receive either too much or too little attention compared to other infectious disease risks. When civilian biodefense is pursued as a biosecurity practice, there is a need to accommodate fear and uncertainty. But there also is a need for public health utility in the prioritization of risks and the allocation of finite resources. If a dual-benefit requirement were imposed, the practical outcome would be the termination of any biodefense activities that afford protection only against nonnatural disease outbreaks. In the United States such activities include the procurement of new smallpox drugs through Project BioShield and the Bio-Watch surveillance project in its entirety. The effort and resources saved could be directed toward establishing or improving activities that can also mitigate naturally occurring infectious disease outbreaks.

The emergence or worsening of infectious disease risks is likely to continue occurring, possibly even more frequently, in the future. Even as the writing of this book was being finished, another episode of heightened political concern about a disease was unfolding. In early 2016 the WHO was reporting that Zika—a mosquito-borne viral disease for which there is no vaccine—was probably the cause of a major increase in cases of microcephaly (small brain) and-or central nervous system malformations in newborn babies. By April there had been over a thousand such cases in Brazil, and Zika-linked cases elsewhere included one reported three months earlier in the United States.[5] Although Zika was not at that time being framed in security terms, some signs were emerging that the disease might come to be regarded as a matter of surpassing importance. On January 26, 2016, for example, President Obama convened a special White House meeting to discuss Zika.[6] The following week, the WHO's director-general announced that Brazil's cluster of Zika-linked microcephaly cases and neurological disorders constituted "a public health emergency of international concern."[7] Obama later announced that $1.9 billion was needed to fund the US response to Zika.[8] If such moves suggest that Zika is a dreaded disease, the basis for that dread is something that warrants further investigation and analysis over time. For now, though, it is clear that Zika is not feared in the same way as the other diseases that are discussed in this book. In contrast to smallpox and plague, for example, infection resulting in death is not the object of concern. Rather, the Zika virus (which usually causes only mild illness in adults) appears to be feared for its potential to inflict deformity and disadvantage on the youngest of human beings.[9] It is conceivable, then, that the freakish spectacle of babies' undersized heads and the associated stigma of diminished mental capacity could become the basis for robust and extraordinary anti-Zika efforts. Thereafter, depending on how governments choose to confront the disease, biosecurity dilemmas might arise.

Wherever dreaded diseases are anticipated or encountered, difficult decisions will be necessary and bold policies may be required. The threatened health of nations can be defended in various ways, but it is important first to be clear about what values are at stake in the practice of biosecurity. For as long as that practice manifests in diverse and conflicting dynamics—protection, proliferation, restriction, freedom, action, overreaction, emphasis, and neglect—biosecurity dilemmas will persist.

NOTES

1. Centers for Disease Control and Prevention, "Zombie Preparedness," Office of Public Health Preparedness and Response, April 10, 2015, http://www.cdc.gov/phpr/zombies.htm.
2. Ali S. Khan, "Preparedness 101: Zombie Apocalypse," Centers for Disease Control and Prevention, May 16, 2011, http://blogs.cdc.gov/publichealthmatters/2011/05/preparedness-101-zombie-apocalypse/.
3. Ibid.
4. See Laura H. Kahn, "Zombie Lessons," *Bulletin of the Atomic Scientists*, July 10, 2013, http://thebulletin.org/zombie-lessons; and Jeremy R. Youde, "Biosurveillance, Human Rights, and the Zombie Plague," in *The Politics of Surveillance and Response*

to Disease Outbreaks: The New Frontier for States and Non-State Actors, ed. Sara E. Davies and Jeremy R. Youde, 58–60 (Farnham, UK: Ashgate, 2015).

5. World Health Organization, "Zika Situation Report," April 14, 2016, http://www. who.int/emergencies/zika-virus/situation-report/14-april-2016/en/.

6. Cheryl Pellerin, "Defense Department Experts to Support HHS with Zika Virus Research," US Department of Defense, January 27, 2016, http://www .defense.gov/News-Article-View/Article/645136/defense-department-experts -to-support-hhs-with-zika-virus-research.

7. World Health Organization, "WHO Director-General Summarizes the Outcome of the Emergency Committee Regarding Clusters of Microcephaly and Guillain-Barré Syndrome," February 1, 2016, http://www.who.int/mediacentre/news /statements/2016/emergency-committee-zika-microcephaly/en/.

8. Barack Obama, "Letter from the President—Zika Virus," White House, February 22, 2016, https://www.whitehouse.gov/the-press-office/2016/02/22/letter-president -zika-virus.

9. World Health Organization, "Zika Virus Fact Sheet," updated April 15, 2016, http://www.who.int/mediacentre/factsheets/zika/en/.

SELECTED BIBLIOGRAPHY

2015 WHO Strategic Response Plan: West Africa Ebola Outbreak. Geneva: World Health Organization, 2015.

A Safer Future: Global Public Health Security in the 21st Century (World Health Report 2007). Geneva: World Health Organization, 2007.

Alcabes, Philip. *Dread: How Fear and Fantasy Have Fueled Epidemics from the Black Death to Avian Flu.* New York: Public Affairs, 2009.

Alibek, Ken. *Biohazard.* London: Arrow, 1999.

Alison, Graham, Robin Cleveland, Steve Rademaker, Tim Roemer, et al. *World at Risk: The Report of the Commission on the Prevention of WMD Proliferation and Terrorism.* New York: Vintage, 2008.

Baldwin, Peter. *Contagion and the State in Europe, 1830–1930.* Cambridge: Cambridge University Press, 2005.

Baram, Michael. "Biotechnological Research on the Most Dangerous Pathogens: Challenges for Risk Governance and Safety Management." *Safety Science* 47, no. 6 (2009): 890–98. http://dx.doi.org/10.1016/j.ssci.2008.10.010.

Battin, Margaret P., Leslie P. Francis, Jay A. Jacobson, et al. *The Patient as Victim and Vector: Ethics and Infectious Disease.* Oxford: Oxford University Press, 2009. http://dx.doi .org/10.1093/acprof:oso/9780195335842.001.0001.

Berger, Kavita M., Carrie Wolinetz, Kari McCarron, et al. *Bridging Science and Security for Biological Research International Science and Security.* Washington, DC: American Association for the Advancement of Science, 2013.

Birn, Anne-Emanuelle. "From Plagues to Peoples: Health on the Modern Global/International Agenda." In *Ashgate Research Companion to the Globalization of Health.* Edited by Ted Schrecker, 39–59. Farnham, UK: Ashgate, 2012.

Boddie, Crystal, Tara Kirk Sell, and Matthew Watson. "Federal Funding for Health Security in FY2015." *Biosecurity and Bioterrorism* 12, no. 4 (2014): 163–77. http://dx.doi .org/10.1089/bsp.2014.0050.

———. "Federal Funding for Health Security in FY2016." *Health Security* 13, no. 3 (2015): 186–206. http://dx.doi.org/10.1089/hs.2015.0017.

Booth, Ken, and Nicholas J. Wheeler. *The Security Dilemma: Fear, Cooperation, and Trust in World Politics.* Basingstoke, UK: Palgrave Macmillan, 2008.

Buzan, Barry, Ole Waever, and Jaap de Wilde. *Security: A New Framework for Analysis.* Boulder, CO: Lynne Rienner, 1998.

Casadevall, Arturo, and Michael J. Imperiale. "Destruction of Microbial Collections in Response to Select Agent and Toxin List Regulations." *Biosecurity and Bioterrorism* 8, no. 2 (2010): 151–54. http://dx.doi.org/10.1089/bsp.2010.0012.

Cello, Jeronimo, Aniko V. Paul, and Eckard Wimmer. "Chemical Synthesis of Poliovirus cDNA: Generation of Infectious Virus in the Absence of Natural Template." *Science* 297, no. 5583 (August 9, 2002): 1016–18. http://dx.doi.org/10.1126/science.1072266.

Chandavarkar, Rajnarayan. "Plague Panic and Epidemic Politics in India, 1896–1914." In *Epidemics and Ideas: Essays on the Historical Perception of Pestilence.* Edited by Terence Ranger and Paul Slack, 203–40. New York: Cambridge University Press, 1992. http://dx.doi.org/10.1017/CBO9780511563645.010.

Clarke, Lee. *Worst Cases: Terror and Catastrophe in the Popular Imagination.* Chicago: University of Chicago Press, 2006.

Cohen, Hillel W., Robert M. Gould, and Victor W. Sidel. "The Pitfalls of Bioterrorism Preparedness: The Anthrax and Smallpox Experiences." *American Journal of Public Health* 94, no. 10 (2004): 1667–71. http://dx.doi.org/10.2105/AJPH.94.10.1667.

Cohen, Jon. "Reinventing Project BioShield." *Science* 333, no. 6047 (September 2, 2011): 1216–18. http://dx.doi.org/10.1126/science.333.6047.1216.

Cohen, Jon, and Martin Enserink. "Rough-and-Tumble behind Bush's Smallpox Policy." *Science* 298, no. 5602 (December 20, 2002): 2312–16. http://dx.doi.org/10.1126/science.298.5602.2312.

Coker, Richard, Marianna Thomas, Karen Lock, et al. "Detention and the Evolving Threat of Tuberculosis: Evidence, Ethics, and Law." *Journal of Law, Medicine, and Ethics* 35, no. 4 (Winter 2007): 609–15. http://dx.doi.org/10.1111/j.1748-720X.2007.00184.x.

Collier, Stephen J., and Andrew Lakoff. "The Problem of Securing Health." In *Biosecurity Interventions: Global Health and Security in Question.* Edited by Andrew Lakoff and Stephen J. Collier, 7–32. New York: Columbia University Press, 2008.

Cooper, Melinda. "Pre-Empting Emergence: The Biological Turn in the War on Terror." *Theory, Culture, and Society* 23, no. 4 (2006): 113–35. http://dx.doi.org/10.1177/0263276406065121.

Daly, Matthew. "Medical Necessity as a Defense for Crimes against Humanity: An Examination of the Molokai Transfers." *Arizona Journal of International and Comparative Law* 24, no. 3 (2007): 645–700.

Davies, Sara E. "Securitizing Infectious Disease." *International Affairs* 84, no. 2 (2008): 295–313. http://dx.doi.org/10.1111/j.1468-2346.2008.00704.x.

DeLaet, Debra L. "Whose Interests Is the Securitization of Health Serving?" In *Routledge Handbook of Global Health Security.* Edited by Simon Rushton and Jeremy Youde, 339–48. New York: Routledge, 2015.

deLisle, Jacques. "SARS, Greater China, and the Pathologies of Globalisation and Transition." *Orbis* 47, no. 4 (2003): 587–604. http://dx.doi.org/10.1016/S0030-4387(03)00076-0.

Deudney, Daniel. *Bounding Power: Republican Security Theory from the Polis to the Global Village.* Princeton: Princeton University Press, 2006.

Dheda, Keertan, and Giovanni B. Migliori. "The Global Rise of Extensively Drug-Resistant Tuberculosis: Is the Time to Bring Back Sanatoria Overdue?" *The Lancet* 379, no. 9817 (February 25, 2012): 773–75. http://dx.doi.org/10.1016/S0140-6736(11)61062-3.

Dhillon, Ranu S., and J. Daniel Kelly. "Community Trust and the Ebola Endgame." *New England Journal of Medicine* 373, no. 9 (2015): 787–89. http://dx.doi.org/10.1056/NEJMp1508413.

Dias, M. Beatrice, Leonardo Reyes-Gonzalez, Francisco M. Veloso, et al. "Effects of the USA PATRIOT Act and the 2002 Bioterrorism Preparedness Act on Select Agent Research in the United States." *Proceedings of the National Academy of Sciences of the United States of America* 107, no. 21 (2010): 9556–61. http://dx.doi.org/10.1073/pnas.0915002107.

Elbe, Stefan. "Should HIV/AIDS Be Securitized? The Ethical Dilemmas of Linking HIV/AIDS and Security." *International Studies Quarterly* 50, no. 1 (2006): 119–44. http://dx.doi.org/10.1111/j.1468-2478.2006.00395.x.

Enemark, Christian. *Disease and Security: Natural Plagues and Biological Weapons in East Asia.* Abingdon, UK: Routledge, 2007. http://dx.doi.org/10.4324/9780203089019.

Fairchild, Amy L., and Eileen A. Tynan. "Policies of Containment: Immigration in the Era of AIDS." *American Journal of Public Health* 84, no. 12 (1994): 2011–22. http://dx.doi.org/10.2105/AJPH.84.12.2011.

Fidler, David P., and Lawrence O. Gostin. *Biosecurity in the Global Age: Biological Weapons, Public Health, and the Rule of Law.* Stanford: Stanford University Press, 2008.

Fischer, Julie E. *Stewardship or Censorship? Balancing Biosecurity, the Public's Health, and the Benefits of Scientific Openness.* Washington, DC: Henry L. Stimson Center, 2006.

Floyd, Rita. "Towards a Consequentialist Evaluation of Security: Bringing Together the Copenhagen and the Welsh Schools of Security Studies." *Review of International Studies* 33, no. 2 (2007): 327–50. http://dx.doi.org/10.1017/S026021050700753X.

Franco, Crystal. "Billions for Biodefense: Federal Agency Biodefense Funding, FY2009–FY2010." *Biosecurity and Bioterrorism* 7, no. 3 (2009): 291–309. http://dx.doi.org/10.1089/bsp.2009.0035.

Franz, David R., Susan A. Ehrlich, Arturo Casadevall, et al. "'The Nuclearization' of Biology Is a Threat to Health and Security." *Biosecurity and Bioterrorism* 7, no. 3 (2009): 243–44. http://dx.doi.org/10.1089/bsp.2009.0047.

Frieden, Thomas R., Jordan W. Tappero, Scott F. Dowell, et al. "Safer Countries through Global Health Security." *Lancet* 383, no. 9919 (March 1, 2014): 764–66. http://dx.doi.org/10.1016/S0140-6736(14)60189-6.

Gainotti, Sabina, Nicola Moran, Carlo Petrini, et al. "Ethical Models Underpinning Responses to Threats to Public Health: A Comparison of Approaches to Communicable Disease Control in Europe." *Bioethics* 22, no. 9 (2008): 466–76. http://dx.doi.org/10.1111/j.1467-8519.2008.00698.x.

Garrett, Laurie. "Biology's Brave New World: The Promise and Perils of the Synbio Revolution." *Foreign Affairs* 6 (November–December 2013): 28–46.

Gensheimer, Kathleen F., Martin I. Meltzer, Alicia S. Postema, et al. "Influenza Pandemic Preparedness." *Emerging Infectious Diseases* 9, no. 12 (2003): 1645–48. http://dx.doi.org/10.3201/eid0912.030289.

Gostin, Lawrence O. "Finding a Space for the Public's Health in Bioterrorism Funding: A Commentary." *American Journal of Bioethics* 5, no. 4 (2005): 45–47. http://dx.doi.org/10.1080/15265160500194220.

Gostin, Lawrence O., and Eric A. Friedman. "A Retrospective and Prospective Analysis of the West African Ebola Virus Disease Epidemic: Robust National Health Systems at the Foundation and an Empowered WHO at the Apex." *Lancet* 385, no. 9980 (May 9, 2015): 1902–9. http://dx.doi.org/10.1016/S0140-6736(15)60644-4.

Gottron, Frank, and Dana A. Shea. *Oversight of High-Containment Biological Laboratories: Issues for Congress*. Washington, DC: Congressional Research Service, 2009.

Graham, Bob, and Jim Talent. "Bioterrorism: Redefining Prevention." *Biosecurity and Bioterrorism* 7, no. 2 (2009): 125–27. http://dx.doi.org/10.1089/bsp.2009.0610.

Gronvall, Gigi Kwik, Joe Fitzgerald, Allison Chamberlain, et al. "High-Containment Biodefense Research Laboratories: Meeting Report and Center Recommendations." *Biosecurity and Bioterrorism* 5, no. 1 (2007): 75–85. http://dx.doi.org/10.1089/bsp.2007.0902.

Henkel, Richard D., Thomas Miller, and Robbin S. Weyant. "Monitoring Select Agent Theft, Loss, and Release Reports in the United States—2004–2010." *Applied Biosafety: Journal of the American Biological Safety Association* 17, no. 4 (2012): 171–80. http://dx.doi.org/10.1177/153567601201700402.

Herfst, Sander, Eefje J. A. Schrauwen, Martin Linster, et al. "Airborne Transmission of Influenza A/H5N1 Virus Between Ferrets." *Science* 336, no. 6088 (June 22, 2012): 1534–41. http://dx.doi.org/10.1126/science.1213362.

Hooker, Claire. "Drawing the Lines: Danger and Risk in the Age of SARS." In *Medicine at the Border: Disease, Globalization and Security, 1850 to the Present*. Edited by Alison Bashford, 179–95. Hampshire, UK: Palgrave Macmillan, 2006.

Hung, Ho-fung. "The Politics of SARS: Containing the Perils of Globalization by More Globalization." *Asian Perspective* 28, no. 1 (2004): 19–44.

Imai, Masaki, Tokiko Watanabe, Masato Hatta, et al. "Experimental Adaptation of an Influenza H5 HA Confers Respiratory Droplet Transmission to a Reassortant H5 HA/H1N1 Virus in Ferrets." *Nature* 486 (June 21, 2012): 420–28.

Jackson, Ronald J., Alistair J. Ramsay, Carina D. Christensen, et al. "Expression of Mouse Interleukin-4 by a Recombinant Ectromelia Virus Suppresses Cytolytic Lymphocyte Responses and Overcomes Genetic Resistance to Mousepox." *Journal of Virology* 75, no. 3 (2001): 1205–10. http://dx.doi.org/10.1128/JVI.75.3.1205-1210.2001.

Jeremias, Gunnar, and Jan van Aken. "Harnessing Global Trade Data for Biological Arms Control." *Nonproliferation Review* 13, no. 2 (2006): 189–209. http://dx.doi.org/10.1080/10736700601012037.

Jervis, Robert. "Cooperation under the Security Dilemma." *World Politics* 30, no. 2 (1978): 167–214. http://dx.doi.org/10.2307/2009958.

Kamradt-Scott, Adam. *Managing Global Health Security: The World Health Organization and Disease Outbreak Control*. Basingstoke, UK: Palgrave Macmillan, 2015. http://dx.doi.org/10.1057/9781137520166.

Kelle, Alexander. "Securitization of International Public Health: Implications for Global Health Governance and the Biological Weapons Prohibition Regime." *Global Governance* 13, no. 2 (2007): 217–35.

Kilbourne, Edwin D. "Influenza Pandemics of the Twentieth Century." *Emerging Infectious Diseases* 12, no. 1 (2006): 9–14. http://dx.doi.org/10.3201/eid1201.051254.

Klotz, Lynn. "Casting a Wider Net for Countermeasure R&D Funding Decision." *Biosecurity and Bioterrorism* 5, no. 4 (2007): 313–8. http://dx.doi.org/10.1089/bsp.2007.0026.

Koblentz, Gregory D. *Living Weapons: Biological Warfare and International Security*. Ithaca, NY: Cornell University Press, 2009.

———. "Biosecurity Reconsidered: Calibrating Biological Threats and Responses." *International Security* 34, no. 4 (2010): 96–132. http://dx.doi.org/10.1162/isec.2010.34.4.96.

————. "From Biodefence to Biosecurity: the Obama Administration's Strategy for Countering Biological Threats." *International Affairs* 88, no. 1 (2012): 131–48. http://dx.doi.org/10.1111/j.1468-2346.2012.01061.x.

Lee, Kelley, and David P. Fidler. "Avian and Pandemic Influenza: Progress and Problems with Global Health Governance." *Global Public Health: An International Journal for Research, Policy and Practice* 2, no. 3 (2007): 215–34. http://dx.doi.org/10.1080/17441690601136947.

Leitenberg, Milton. "Distinguishing Offensive from Defensive Biological Weapons Research." *Critical Reviews in Microbiology* 29, no. 3 (2003): 223–57. http://dx.doi.org/10.1080/713610450.

————. *Assessing the Biological Weapons and Bioterrorism Threat.* Carlisle, PA: Strategic Studies Institute, 2005.

Lentzos, Filippa. "Hard to Prove." *Nonproliferation Review* 18, no. 3 (2011): 571–82. http://dx.doi.org/10.1080/10736700.2011.618662.

McInnes, Colin, and Kelley Lee. "Health, Security and Foreign Policy." *Review of International Studies* 32, no. 1 (2006): 5–23. http://dx.doi.org/10.1017/S0260210506006905.

Meselson, Matthew, Jeanne Guillemin, Martin Hugh-Jones, et al. "The Sverdlovsk Anthrax Outbreak of 1979." *Science* 266, no. 5188 (November 18, 1994): 1202–8. http://dx.doi.org/10.1126/science.7973702.

Miller, Judith, Stephen Engelberg, and William Broad. *Germs: The Ultimate Weapon.* London: Simon and Schuster, 2001.

Miller, Seumas, and Michael J. Selgelid. *Ethical and Philosophical Consideration of the Dual-Use Dilemma in the Biological Sciences.* Dordrecht, Netherlands: Springer, 2008. http://dx.doi.org/10.1007/978-1-4020-8312-9.

National Research Council. *Beyond "Fortress America": National Security Controls on Science and Technology in a Globalized World.* Washington, DC: National Academies Press, 2009.

————. *Biotechnology Research in an Age of Terrorism.* Washington, DC: National Academy of Sciences, 2004.

————. *Globalization, Biosecurity, and the Future of the Life Sciences.* Washington, DC: National Academies Press, 2006.

————. *Responsible Research with Biological Select Agents and Toxins.* Washington, DC: National Academies Press, 2009.

————. *Review of the Scientific Approaches Used during the FBI's Investigation of the 2001 Anthrax Letters.* Washington, DC: National Academies Press, 2011.

————. *Science and Security in a Post 9/11 World: A Report Based on Regional Discussions between the Science and Security Communities.* Washington, DC: National Academies Press, 2007.

Nuzzo, Jennifer B., Anita J. Cicero, Richard Waldhorn, et al. "Travel Bans Will Increase the Damage Wrought by Ebola." *Biosecurity and Bioterrorism* 12, no. 6 (2014): 306–9. http://dx.doi.org/10.1089/bsp.2014.1030.

O'Manique, Colleen. "Global Health and the Human Security Agenda." In *Ashgate Research Companion to the Globalization of Health.* Edited by Ted Schrecker, 151–68. Farnham, UK: Ashgate, 2012.

Ouagrham-Gormley, Sonia Ben. "Barriers to Bioweapons: Intangible Obstacles to Proliferation." *International Security* 36, no. 4 (2012): 80–114. http://dx.doi.org/10.1162/ISEC_a_00077.

Parmet, Wendy. "Legal Power and Legal Rights—Isolation and Quarantine in the Case of Drug-Resistant Tuberculosis." *New England Journal of Medicine* 357, no. 5 (2007): 433–35. http://dx.doi.org/10.1056/NEJMp078133.

Patrone, Daniel, David Resnik, and Lisa Chin. "Biosecurity and the Review and Publication of Dual Use Research of Concern." *Biosecurity and Bioterrorism* 10, no. 3 (2012): 290–98. http://dx.doi.org/10.1089/bsp.2012.0011.

Peterson, Susan. "Epidemic Disease and National Security." *Security Studies* 12, no. 2 (2002): 43–81. http://dx.doi.org/10.1080/0963-640291906799.

Pinto, Andrew D., Anne-Emanuelle Birn, and Ross E. G. Upshur. "The Context of Global Health Ethics." In *An Introduction to Global Health Ethics.* Edited by Andrew D. Pinto and Ross E. G. Upshur, 3–15. New York: Routledge, 2013.

Price-Smith, Andrew T. *Contagion and Chaos: Disease, Ecology, and National Security in the Era of Globalization.* Cambridge, MA: MIT Press, 2009.

———. *The Health of Nations: Infectious Disease, Environmental Change, and Their Effects on National Security and Development.* Cambridge: MIT Press, 2002.

Rappert, Brian. *Biotechnology, Security, and the Search for Limits: An Inquiry into Research and Methods.* Basingstoke, UK: Palgrave Macmillan, 2007. http://dx.doi.org/10.1057/9780230223158.

———. "Codes of Conduct and Biological Weapons: An In-Process Assessment." *Biosecurity and Bioterrorism* 5, no. 2 (2007): 145–54. http://dx.doi.org/10.1089/bsp.2007.0003.

Richards, Stephanie L., Victoria C. Pompei, and Alice Anderson. "BSL-3 Laboratory Practices in the United States: Comparison of Select Agent and Non-Select Agent Facilities." *Biosecurity and Bioterrorism* 12, no. 1 (2014): 1–7. http://dx.doi.org/10.1089/bsp.2013.0060.

Roberts, Marc J., and Michael R. Reich. "Ethical Analysis in Public Health." *Lancet* 359, no. 9311 (March 23, 2002): 1055–59. http://dx.doi.org/10.1016/S0140-6736(02)08097-2.

Roffey, Roger, and Chandré Gould. "Preventing Misuse of the Life Sciences: The Need to Improve Biodefense Transparency and Accountability in the BWC." *Nonproliferation Review* 18, no. 3 (2011): 557–69. http://dx.doi.org/10.1080/10736700.2011.618659.

Rushton, Simon. "Global Health Security: Security for Whom? Security from What?" *Political Studies* 59, no. 4 (2011): 779–96. http://dx.doi.org/10.1111/j.1467-9248.2011.00919.x.

Schell, Heather. "Outburst! A Chilling True Story about Emerging-Virus Narratives and Pandemic Social Change." *Configurations* 5, no. 1 (1997): 93–133. http://dx.doi.org/10.1353/con.1997.0006.

Schwellenbach, Nick. "Biodefense: A Plague of Researchers." *Bulletin of the Atomic Scientists* 61, no. 3 (2005): 14–16.

Selgelid, Michael J. "Ethics and Infectious Disease." *Bioethics* 19, no. 3 (2005): 272–89. http://dx.doi.org/10.1111/j.1467-8519.2005.00441.x.

———. "A Moderate Pluralist Approach to Public Health Policy and Ethics." *Public Health Ethics* 2, no. 2 (2009): 195–205. http://dx.doi.org/10.1093/phe/php018.

Selgelid, Michael J., and Lorna Weir. "Reflections on the Synthetic Production of Poliovirus." *Bulletin of the Atomic Scientists* 66, no. 3 (2010): 1–9. http://dx.doi.org/10.2968/066003001.

Sell, Tara Kirk, and Matthew Watson. "Federal Agency Biodefense Funding, FY2013–FY2014." *Biosecurity and Bioterrorism* 11, no. 3 (2013): 196–216. http://dx.doi.org/10.1089/bsp.2013.0047.

Slovic, Paul, Baruch Fischhoff, and Sarah Lichtenstein. "Facts and Fears: Understanding Perceived Risk." In *Societal Risk Assessment: How Safe is Safe Enough?* Edited by Richard C. Schwing and Walter A. Albers, 181–216. New York: Plenum, 1980. http://dx.doi.org/10.1007/978-1-4899-0445-4_9.

Smith, Charles B., Margaret P. Battin, Jay A. Jacobsen, et al. "Are There Characteristics of Infectious Diseases That Raise Special Ethical Issues?" In *Ethics and Infectious Disease*. Edited by Michael J. Selgelid, Margaret P. Battin, and Charles B. Smith, 20–34. Malden, UK: Blackwell, 2006.

Stern, Jessica. "Dreaded Risks and the Control of Biological Weapons." *International Security* 27, no. 3 (2002–2003): 89–123. http://dx.doi.org/10.1162/01622880260553642.

St. John, Ronald K., Arlene King, Dick de Jong, et al. "Border Screening for SARS." *Emerging Infectious Diseases* 11, no. 1 (2005): 6–10. http://dx.doi.org/10.3201/eid1101.040835.

Stuckler, David, and Martin McKee. "Five Metaphors about Global-Health Policy." *Lancet* 372, no. 9633 (July 12, 2008): 95–97. http://dx.doi.org/10.1016/S0140-6736(08)61013-2.

Sunstein, Cass R. "Terrorism and Probability Neglect." *Journal of Risk and Uncertainty* 26, no. 2/3 (2003): 121–36. http://dx.doi.org/10.1023/A:1024111006336.

Tang, Shiping. "Fear in International Politics: Two Positions." *International Studies Review* 10, no. 3 (2008): 451–71. http://dx.doi.org/10.1111/j.1468-2486.2008.00800.x.

Taubenberger, Jeffery K., Ann H. Reid, Raina M. Lourens, et al. "Characterization of the 1918 Influenza Virus Polymerase Genes." *Nature* 437, no. 7060 (October 6, 2005): 889–93. http://dx.doi.org/10.1038/nature04230.

Thucydides. *History of the Peloponnesian War*. Translated by Rex Warner. Harmondsworth, UK: Penguin, 1954.

Tucker, Jonathan B. *Scourge: The Once and Future Threat of Smallpox*. New York: Atlantic Monthly Press, 2001.

———. "Biological Threat Assessment: Is the Cure Worse Than the Disease?" *Arms Control Today* 34 (2004): 13–19.

Tumpey, Terrence M., Christopher F. Basler, Patricia V. Aguilar, et al. "Characterization of the Reconstructed 1918 Spanish Influenza Pandemic Virus." *Science* 310, no. 5745 (2005): 77–80. http://dx.doi.org/10.1126/science.1119392.

UN Commission on Human Rights. "Siracusa Principles on the Limitation and Derogation Provisions in the International Covenant on Civil and Political Rights." *Human Rights Quarterly* 7, no. 1 (1985): 3–14. http://dx.doi.org/10.2307/762035.

Upshur, Ross E. G. "Principles for the Justification of Public Health Intervention." *Canadian Journal of Public Health* 93 (2002): 101–3.

Verweij, Marcel, and Angus Dawson. "Shutting Up Infected Houses: Infectious Disease Control, Past and Present." *Public Health Ethics* 3, no. 1 (2010): 1–3. http://dx.doi.org/10.1093/phe/phq008.

Vogel, Kathleen M. *Phantom Menace or Looming Danger?: A New Framework for Assessing Bioweapons Threats*. Baltimore, MD: Johns Hopkins University Press, 2013.

Wald, Priscilla. *Contagious: Cultures, Carriers, and the Outbreak Narrative*. London: Duke University Press, 2008.

Watson, Scott. "Back Home, Safe and Sound: The Public and Private Production of Insecurity." *International Political Sociology* 5, no. 2 (2011): 160–77. http://dx.doi .org/10.1111/j.1749-5687.2011.00127.x.

Wein, Lawrence M., and Yifan Liu. "Analyzing a Bioterror Attack on the Food Supply: The Case of Botulinum Toxin in Milk." *Proceedings of the National Academy of Sciences of the United States of America* 102, no. 28 (2005): 9984–89. http://dx.doi .org/10.1073/pnas.0408526102.

Weir, Lorna. "Inventing Global Health Security, 1994–2005." In *Routledge Handbook of Global Health Security*. Edited by Simon Rushton and Jeremy Youde, 18–31. New York: Routledge, 2015.

Wheelis, Mark, and Malcolm Dando. "Back to Bioweapons?" *Bulletin of the Atomic Scientists* 59, no. 1 (January–February 2003): 41–46. http://dx.doi.org/10.1080/00963 402.2003.11460645.

World Health Organization. *Ethical Considerations in Developing a Public Health Response to Pandemic Influenza*. Report No. WHO/CDS/EPR/GIP/2007.2. Geneva: World Health Organization, 2007.

———. *Fighting Disease, Fostering Development*. World Health Report 1996. Geneva: World Health Organization, 1996.

———. *Global Tuberculosis Report 2014*. Geneva: World Health Organization, 2014.

———. *Guidance on Ethics of Tuberculosis Prevention, Care and Control*. Report No. WHO/HTM/TB/2010.16. Geneva: World Health Organization, 2010.

———. *International Health Regulations (2005)*. 2nd ed. Geneva: World Health Organization, 2008.

———. *Pandemic Influenza Preparedness Framework for the Sharing of Influenza Viruses and Access to Vaccines and Other Benefits*. Geneva: World Health Organization, 2011.

———. *Reducing Risks, Promoting Healthy Life (World Health Report 2002)*. Geneva: World Health Organization, 2002.

———. *WHO Global Influenza Preparedness Plan: The Role of WHO and Recommendations for National Measures before and during Pandemics (WHO/CDS/CSR/GIP/2005.5)*. Geneva: World Health Organization, 2005.

World Health Organization Writing Group. "Nonpharmaceutical Interventions for Pandemic Influenza, International Measures." *Emerging Infectious Diseases* 12, no. 1 (2006): 81–87. http://dx.doi.org/10.3201/eid1201.051370.

Wolfers, Arnold. " 'National Security' as an Ambiguous Symbol." *Political Science Quarterly* 67, no. 4 (1952): 481–502. http://dx.doi.org/10.2307/2145138.

Youde, Jeremy R. "Biosurveillance, Human Rights, and the Zombie Plague." In *The Politics of Surveillance and Response to Disease Outbreaks: The New Frontier for States and Non-State Actors*. Edited by Sara E. Davies and Jeremy R. Youde, 857–69. Farnham, UK: Ashgate, 2015.

Zimmer, Shanta M., and Donald S. Burke. "Historical Perspective—Emergence of Influenza A (H1N1) Viruses." *New England Journal of Medicine* 361, no. 3 (2009): 279–85. http://dx.doi.org/10.1056/NEJMra0904322.

Zylberman, Patrick. "Civilizing the State: Borders, Weak States, and International Health in Modern Europe." In *Medicine at the Border: Disease, Globalization and Security, 1850 to the Present*. Edited by Alison Bashford, 21–40. Hampshire, UK: Palgrave Macmillan, 2006.

INDEX

ABOUT THE AUTHOR

CHRISTIAN ENEMARK is Professor of International Relations at the University of Southampton in the United Kingdom. He has also held positions at Aberystwyth University, the Australian National University, and the University of Sydney. His previous books are *Disease and Security: Natural Plagues and Biological Weapons in East Asia* (Routledge, 2007); *Ethics and Security Aspects of Infectious Disease Control: Interdisciplinary Perspectives* (Ashgate, 2012); and *Armed Drones and the Ethics of War: Military Virtue in a Post-Heroic Age* (Routledge, 2014). He has published articles in journals including *Bioethics, Ethics & International Affairs, Health Policy and Planning, Nonproliferation Review, Security Studies*, and *Survival*, and he serves on the international editorial board of *Contemporary Security Policy*.

CPSIA information can be obtained
at www.ICGtesting.com
Printed in the USA
LVOW03*2121160717
541290LV00007B/128/P